FACE IT

Five Essential Elements for Living Beautifully
Tips for Beauties Over 50

by GAIL SAGEL

Author of Making FACES Beautiful®

Contents:

"I know so many cosmetic executives, and Gail really is at the top of her game."

Judy Goss – CEO of Over40Females, Former Editor of *Cosmopolitan and More Magazine*

"I love your Brush-On Liquid Mineral so much. I get so many samples, but always go back to yours!

Janene Mascarella – Beauty Director *Bella Magazine* and beauty + health consultant at *PARADE Magazine*

"Gail is realistic and understands anyone who has an active busy lifestyle."

Kathy McShane – Managing Director of Ladies Who Launch

"Working with Gail is like working with an artist."

Catherine Frels – Actress

"Thank you for making such great products! You definitely get women. Makes getting my face ready for the day so much easier!"

Kimberly Harbour – Beauty Blogger

Welcome to FACE IT, a book that illustrates my most intimate beauty and lifestyle secrets. My goal is to facilitate beauty by making it easy to achieve and maintain, inside and out. Every topic within these pages comes from decades of life experiences and conversations with my clients – women just like you.

When it comes to all elements essential for inner and outer beauty, women's beauty – eyebrows, makeup, hair, skincare, diet, exercise – let this manual be your guide. If you can master just one aspect of your face, you will have achieved meaningful success. Mastering all three major areas – skin, eyes and lips – you can be forever transformed.

To illustrate the importance of mastering even one beauty area, let me share an ongoing example. Over the years, I've had the opportunity to shape eyebrows in many unique and sometimes awkward situations. For example, at my annual mammogram check up, my bare breasts squeezed like lemons into the machine's cold clamps, my nurse technician exclaims, "wow, what great brows you have!" Not, breasts, but brows. Over the next half hour, we are engaged in an intense conversation about everything eyebrow, from tweezing to trimming to filling. While I got a new client for life, I was happier to hear my mammogram came back normal.

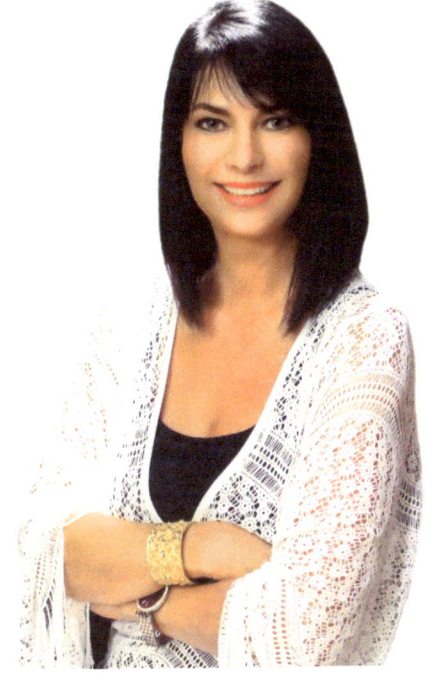

In addition to my expertise in brows, I am sought after in all areas of the face, helping women attain enhanced beauty easily and quickly. Encountering women everywhere: at my studio, as a national speaker for Over 40 Females (my favorite networking group), and even in my doctor's office, I have occasion to discuss beauty issues and concerns. What I hear over and over again – is the challenge women have in living a contemporary busy lifestyle, while sustaining a manageable beauty regimen that doesn't overwhelm their time constraints.

My goal is to help you be the most beautiful you, every day, morning, noon and night. For me, it's never just about the makeup, it is about making our entire lifestyle easier.

Be beautiful,

Gail Sagel

FACE IT – We're beautiful at every age, but often don't appreciate how good we looked in our youth until we look back at pictures. But with my eyebrow advice and beauty tips, you'll be feeling fresh and pretty in no time.

Let's start with something often ignored, but perhaps the most important part of the face, the EYEBROWS!

A few weeks ago, I hosted an eyebrow makeover party at my Faces Beautiful® studio for 10 eyebrow clients, all fabulous and over 50. Why this group? Well, younger women don't ask for my stay-young tricks nearly as often as my mature customers. My baby boomer clients understand and appreciate the importance of a clean, well-shaped brow. Frustrated with sparse brows or irritated by long-wiry hairs, after our makeover, my clients feel as though they've had a mini facelift after a good brow shaping and brow filling.

It was like a little Girls' Night Out party. I put together a wonderful spread of fresh vegetables, hummus, black bean salsa, gluten free chips, and several bottles of red and white wine. I asked the very talented top makeup artist, Erica Durso, to join me and I invited the head of Bridgeport High School photography department, Brian Schmitt, to photograph the Before and After makeovers. I asked these women to come either with no makeup or however they had been made up prior that day. It was such a successful evening that it inspired me to write this book.

At a time when advertising is directed to the millennials, why am I focused on reaching baby boomers? Female baby boomers are one of the largest sectors of American generational groups. Studies show that this group is living longer than ever, and that as a group we spend the most money—especially when it comes to cosmetics and beauty.

When I was a junior in college, my father asked me what I wanted to do when I grew up. I told him I wanted to work in skincare and cosmetics. With a raised eyebrow, he asked me, "Why?" I responded that we were going to be the first generation to live to 100 and we were going to need all of the help we could get. Daddy laughed. He clearly did not think that was a good career path for me. Instead he suggested that I put my analytical mind to work on Wall Street. Well, I did and that was not a happy ever after ending. I decided to change my path, realizing that beauty was my calling, and I've never looked back since.

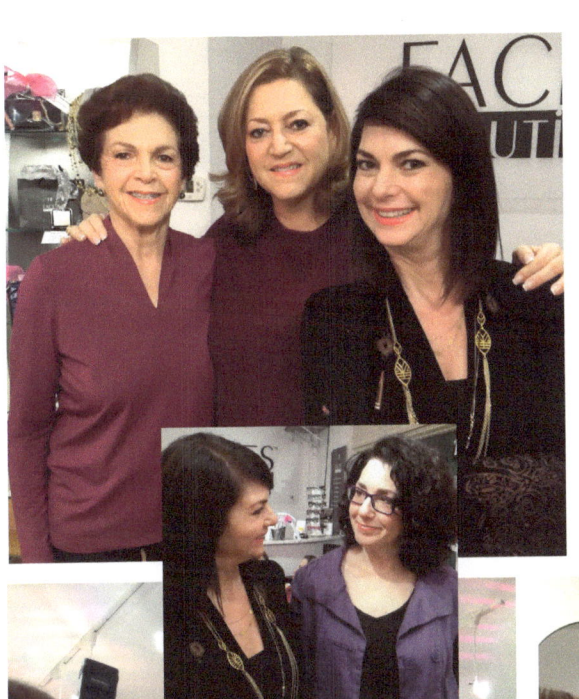
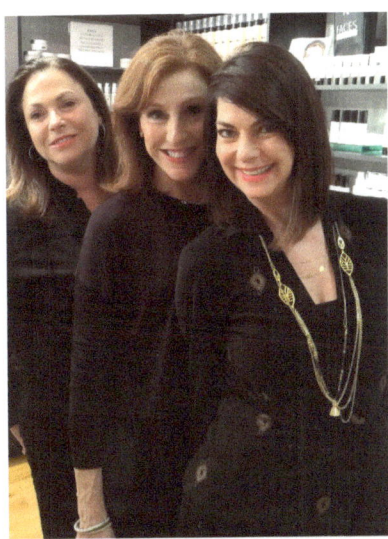
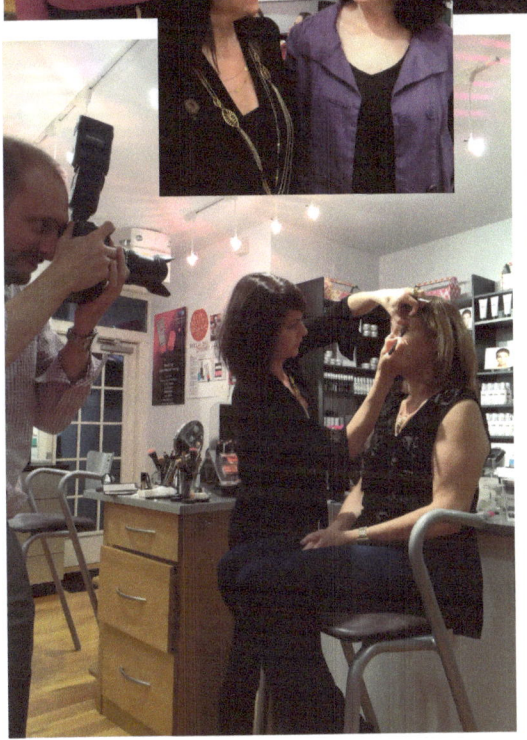
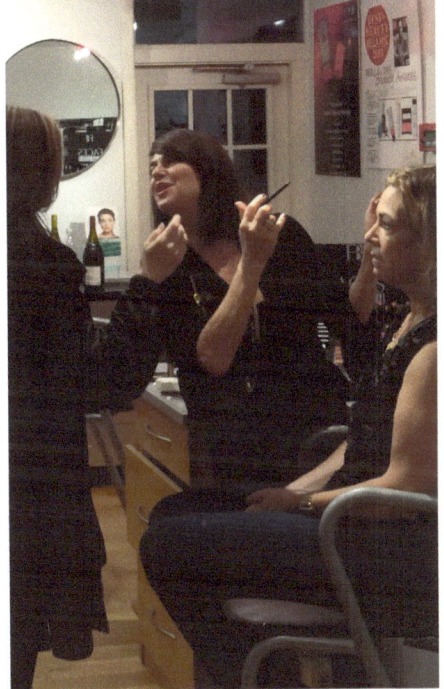
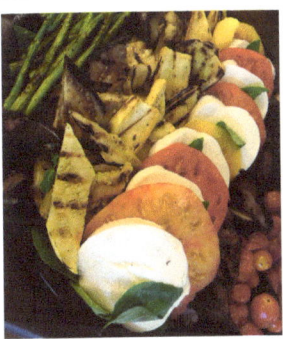
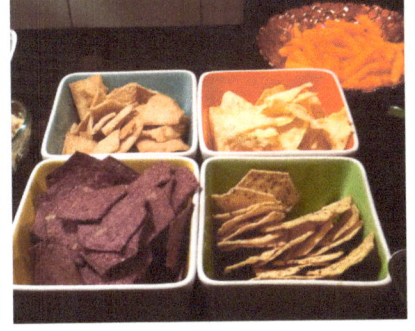
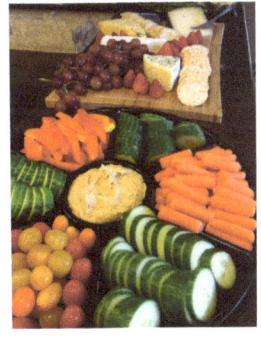

This book is about sharing my beauty tips and secrets. You know that feeling you get when you have a fresh haircut or blowout and you just feel prettier? Hence, the success of blow dry salons. I don't know if I can say specifically that anyone's head actually turns when I step out after my hair is done, but I do feel more positive energy from the world around me. Is it that I look prettier? Or is it that my positive energy is elevated and therefore the world reacts more positively back towards me? Either way, my day, even if only for that moment, is changed for the better. This is the philosophy I want to share with you.

Of course, this age can be a very difficult time for any number of reasons, but it's our approach to these challenges, which defines us. Every stage of womanhood gives us a full plate of obstacles to handle. So why should this decade be any different? In this stage we're dealing with the emotional and physical aspects of menopause. Perhaps we may also be coping with financial issues, personal money management, children leaving the nest, college expenses, stressful career changes, aging parents, grand parenting, and pursuing new career paths. For me, I've certainly been challenged by family illness, divorce, single parenting, career transitions, and financial struggles, just to name a few on my pretty long list of life's curve balls.

"Ladies, you better spend as much on your face as you spend on your shoes because in a few years, if your face doesn't look good, then who's gonna bother to look at your shoes!"

But, this is also an exciting and adventurous time. In talking with friends and clients, who are 50+, we all agree that we are enjoying a new chapter; whether we are appreciating being empty nesters, discovering new-found intimacy with our spouse, or entering the dating world for the first time in decades, this stage can be invigorating. Everything is new again and anything is possible.

My last book, *Making Faces Beautiful*, addressed women of all ages. It spoke to the "me" generation. This book is tailored to my baby boomer contemporaries.

In this manual focused on us 50+ girls, I will share how to bring back your brows, plump up your skin, minimize fine lines, make your eyes pop, (even if your lids are "crepe-y") and achieve full, voluptuous lips.

In addition to acknowledging Erica and Brian, I'd like to take this opportunity to thank others who were critical in completing this endeavor.

- I'd like to credit Sabrina Diamond and Emma Lederer for helping to edit and organize this book. Emma is a creative communications major at Penn State and Sabrina is a bright and meticulous Fordham University student.
- Ken Kast, photographer and photographic expert, whose countless hours and dedication provided this book its special glow.
- Marla Aaron Wapner, a true friend and supporter, who was critical in all aspects of the text and editorial.
- I'm eternally grateful to the person who knows better than anyone -- how to dot my i's and cross my t's and do it with love -- my brilliant and talented daughter, Sarah J Cohen.
- Cindy Schreibman, a creative, marketing, and editing guru without whose guidance and focus on my brand development might never have made this book come to fruition.

When I apply their makeup, women always ask about my secrets in making them look beautiful. My clients love hearing my tips on health and skin care, nutrition and healthy recipes (what I'm eating and cooking), and fitness (my latest exercise routine). I'm always happy to share with them what I know. As a proud member of the 50+ club, I'm now going to share my secrets, antidotes, advice, and witticisms with you.

Five Essential Elements for Living Beautifully

There are Five Essential Elements for Living Beautifully, which will keep you 50+ ladies looking fabulous. If you want to transform to ageless beauty, then get to know my 5 E's.

The Five Essential Elements for Living Beautifully:

1. Exfoliate

2. Eyes

3. Exercise

4. Eat

5. Energy

EXFOLIATE

The First Essential Element for Living Beautifully

Wash Those Wrinkles Right Off of Your Face...

Before I share my many makeup and eyebrow tips, I have to say that your biggest beauty consideration should be your skin and getting it in tip-top condition. The better your skin, the less makeup you'll need. In fact, keeping your skin freshly exfoliated and well hydrated is the secret. Many beauty lines encourage you to hydrate and moisturize. Well, I have a different theory. I believe you should exfoliate more than you hydrate.

Exfoliation does more than just whisk away complexion-dulling dead skin cells. Exfoliating increases cell turnover to reveal newer, healthier skin cells, plus it decreases blackheads and breakouts, minimizes hyperpigmentation and fine lines, reduces the appearance of large pores, and imparts an all-over healthy glow. It also helps hydration. Cells transitioning from below the skin's surface to the top layer bring with them essential lipids and moisture. Serum and moisturizers are better absorbed into skin that's not blocked by layers of dead cells and dirt. Regular exfoliating of your face will also help your makeup go on smoother and more evenly.

While regular skin cleansing is clearly beneficial, exfoliating your face on a regular basis can improve the results of your skin care routine and help rejuvenate your skin. Whether you have dry, normal, oily, or sensitive skin, exfoliation can bring new life to your complexion. You should do some type of exfoliation every day, using various different exfoliators, and then moisturize just enough to plump up your skin and leave it dewy.

> **"You get wiser as you get older; age wisely too."**

Exfoliating your skin is a bit like exercising your body. There are many different types of exfoliators, just as there are many types of exercise, from cardio to toning. Most exercises share a common goal, which is to increase oxygen flow and circulation and create tone. We all know the expression, "No pain, no gain," which means that the following day you will ache a bit. It means you actually pushed your body to a new level. Exfoliation for your skin is actually quite similar. Just like exercise there are many types of exfoliators. I put them into two groups. There are physical exfoliators, like facial scrubs, microdermabrasion, or washcloths. (These products or materials move or remove the skin.)

10

Then there are chemical exfoliators, products with active ingredients like alpha hydroxyls, botanical enzymes, lactic acids, vitamin A, and Retin-A (tretinoin). (These exfoliators gently break up the top layer of skin to allow it to slough and peel off.) A combination of using both types of exfoliators will constantly keep dead skin cells off your skin.

"If it scares you, it might be a good thing to try."

Removing the top layer of your skin this frequently will actually fool your skin into thinking that your skin cells are turning over at a faster pace, just like when you were younger. Skin cells that turn over faster need less moisturizer, because the skin is more supple. Realize that your skin, the largest organ in your body, produces oil on demand. Bodies are created to respond and recalculate based upon the required task, much like when a new mother nurses, her body produces milk on her baby's demand. The moment that mother begins to supplement, the body will create less milk. So, if you are giving your skin a ton of moisture, the body sends the message that it doesn't need to create the moisture and turn the skin cells over.

The trick is to find the balance, and for every woman it's different for how much you can exfoliate, force the skin cell turnover, and then give just enough moisture to hydrate without saturation. So whether you use a wash cloth when cleansing, a daily facial scrub, apply a retinol cream several times a week, have microdermabrasion or facial peels several times a month – nothing will make your skin glow more than constantly removing the dead skin cell buildup.

Karen

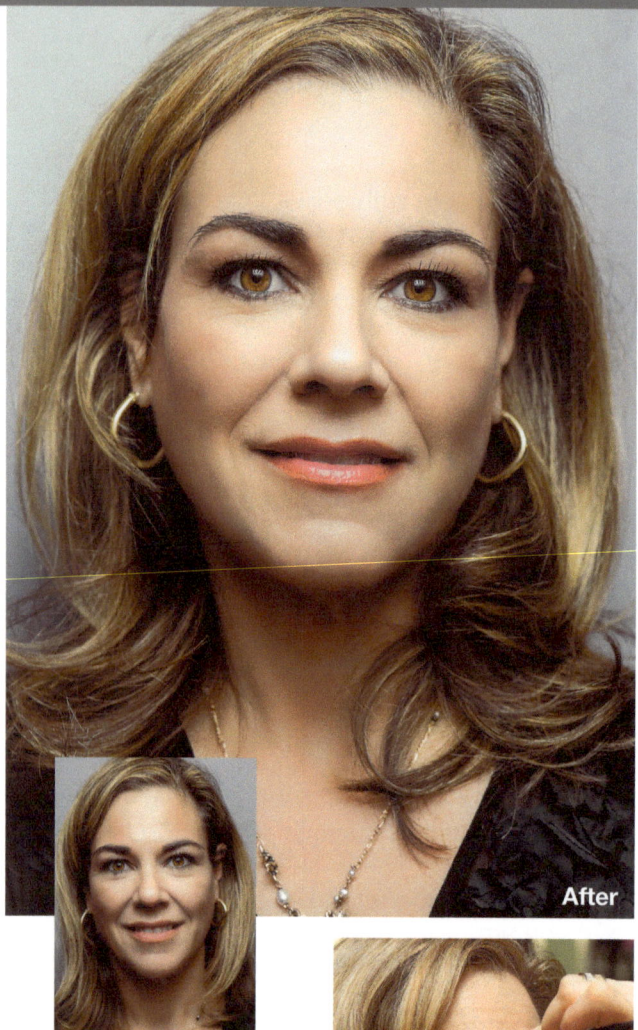

After

Before

Karen gets gorgeous...

I started with a toner to refresh her skin. Next, I used a lightweight moisturizer on her face, and then followed up by applying a liquid mineral makeup. I used the attached foundation brush to blend it all over her face, under her chin, and into her neck just a bit.

Karen's brows were a little over-waxed between her nose. The angle is very straight. In order to correct this, I used a brow balm and I drew on the ends in an angle to her nose. I used a small angle eye-shadow brush to do this. Once I had the angle in place, I dipped the brush into a black eye shadow and went over the balm very lightly for a fuller, deeper look.

For her eyes, I used the a palette of neutral brown eye shadows using the **Reverse Nude Eye Shadow Technique** and added an extra layer of gel eye liner.

- **LID** – Apply a dark brown eyeshadow on the eyelid
- **CONTOUR** – Contour the eyelid with a medium brown eye shadow
- **LINER** – Wet your eyeliner brush, and line the eyes with a dark brown eye shadow
- **GEL LINER** – Apply black liner on the top and bottom, blend with the dark brown eye shadow. Apply a blue liner on the inner water line.
- **MASCARA** – Apply black mascara to top and bottom lashes.

To pop her cheeks and accentuate her eyes, I used my **Bronze & Blush Face Lift Technique**. I began with bronzer and used it sparingly, only applying a small amount under her cheekbones. After this, I mixed together a pink blush and a coral blush and applied this just above the bronzer.

For Karen's lips, I chose a warm, coral toned lipstick. I didn't use any lip-liner, but I finished off her look using a cranberry colored lip gloss.

Karen, fabulous and newly 50, was my first makeover of the night. She could barely fit us in her busy schedule. She joined us right after work and had plans to go out immediately after her makeover. Like most of us, she packs a lot into every day and every night. However, applying makeup doesn't have to be difficult or time consuming.

I want to teach Karen how to accentuate her lovely dark eyebrows. I'm also going to show Karen how to play up her eyes, since she loves lots of black eyeliner. In addition to accentuating Karen's eyes and eyebrows, I'm going to show her how to frame her eyes with shadow and blush too.

I loved having my makeup done by a professional. It definitely taught me some tricks that I now use in my everyday routine. I was so happy that I got a great look for every day that I could re- create myself.

Karen

Tips to Even Your Skin Tone

We all know what hyper-pigmentation is – unattractive. Even if your skin is healthy, past sun damage or medications can leave dark marks on your skin. You don't have to have these spots. You can remove and lighten this discoloration. The first thing is that your skin must be well exfoliated. That is key. Think of it this way: If your skin is not well exfoliated, then whatever product you're using, no matter how effective, just won't penetrate. Imagine if you're wearing a pair of rubber gloves and you put hand cream on your hands. Is it penetrating to your hands? No. The only way for the hand cream to get to your hands is to remove the rubber gloves and the only way for a lightening product to get into your skin is to constantly remove the dead skin cells. And, you can't do it just once. You have to keep removing the skin cells. Women who come in for microdermabrasion once a year always ask me if that's enough. No, it's not enough. You must have an at home exfoliation routine too. So, how do you remove hyper-pigmentation? If you ask your dermatologist, she'll probably recommend a product with hydroquinone. It can work; it's not necessarily my favorite. It's also not on the EU list of cosmetics. Cosmetics in the European Union are more strictly regulated than in the U.S. Hydroquinone doesn't meet the EU safety requirements. I tend to prefer lightening with ingredients that are more natural and a better way to deactivate the melanin in your skin.

Here's my lightening ingredient list:

1. **Kojic Acid**
   Derived from fungal species, this ingredient is chemically related to hydroquinone and helps to inhibit tyrosinase, which is an enzyme involved in melanin production. Kojic acid is also an antioxidant, so it can help protect from future free radical damage that may worsen hyperpigmentation.

2. **Licorice Root**
   Related to beans and peas, licorice root produces an extract that reduces inflammation and helps to naturally lighten hyperpigmentation. It contains an active compound called glabridin that inhibits the enzyme that causes skin to darken in response to sun exposure. Glabridin decreases the production of melanin, and over time will lighten scars and dark spots.

3. **Green Tea**
   Green tea helps inhibit tyrosinase, reducing melanin production.

4. **Kiwi**
   Like kojic acid, kiwi fruit extract has been found to help inhibit the production of tyrosinase. Like most fruit extracts, kiwi is also rich in protective antioxidants.

5. **Turmeric**
   As a powerful anti-inflammatory and antioxidant, it can inhibit the production of melanin to even out skin tone.

Three More Tips

1. I like to add a vitamin C serum, just after exfoliation. Vitamin C is a wonderful way of waking up the collagen in your skin. Collagen is like the rubber bands of your skin and we want to keep that tone.

2. I take my makeup off every day. I don't sleep with it. Yuk.

3. I use sunscreen daily on my face, neck, and hands. You don't want new sunspots, especially when you're working so hard to remove the ones you have now.

Now here's a simple trick to have soft, supple skin on your body too!

Every day, before I shower, I use a dry brush and brush my entire body – feet, legs, arms, butt, breasts, neck. When I'm finished showering, and still wet, I spray oil on my body. Then I towel off. I keep a spray bottle in my shower filled with almond oil or EVOO and sometimes I'll rub on coconut oil too.

Let's Talk Face Makeup

Once you're well exfoliated, your skin is ready to go. Remember – less is more. Many women make the mistake of trying to cover wrinkles with heavy foundations and powders. It just makes you look worse. Less is actually more when it comes to downplaying your facial flaws. A face full of heavy foundation only highlights wrinkles. Instead of a foundation, try a tinted moisturizer or a BB cream, (aka beauty balm cream.) They both provide lighter coverage, won't settle into your wrinkles, and won't cling to facial hairs that pop up on some postmenopausal women's faces.

> ## "You just haven't lived 'til you've had your makeup done."

You can also achieve a smoother finish by applying a primer in between your moisturizer and your foundation/tinted moisturizer. A primer will help your makeup last all day. Applying a layer of primer between your skin and makeup will help your eye shadow and foundation glide on flawlessly -- and most importantly -- stay put and last all day. I recommend primers wherever you are putting makeup.

Eye primers should be used for eye shadows and face primer for your face. In the makeovers here, I used an eye shadow primer on everyone. I didn't include that in my steps for each woman, as it was redundant. I didn't use face primers on everyone, because some of the products have primers built in.

Carol gets glammed up…

I began by smoothing and evening her skin tone using a hydrating primer and our Brush-On Makeup. Using the attached brush, I blended her face, under her chin and into her neck.

As a natural part of getting older, Carol's brows have thinned and in some places disappeared. I focused especially on filling in places that were sparse using a brow balm, applying it with an angle brush.

For her eyes, I kept things simple. Even though it looks like Carol has no eye shadow on, it's actually a very nude eyelid. I applied different shades of nude eye shadows using my **Side "V" Eye Shadow Technique** in order to achieve a very natural look.

- **LINE** – Apply a black liner on top and on bottom
- **LID** – Use a neutral light cream eye shadow
- **"V"** – Apply Light Beige "V"
- **POP** – Apply Light Cream Sheen eye shadow
- **MASCARA** – Use mascara on the top lashes.

To pop her cheeks I used my **Bronze & Blush Face Lift Technique.**

- **BRONZER** – Apply bronzer under the chin, jaw, and over the neck area.
- **BLUSH** – Pop a touch of Pink blush just above bronzer.
- **HIGHLIGHTER** – Use a highlighter just above the blush, blending it into the eye area.

For Carol's lips, I decided to go with a bold red color. Carol has a great mouth and wears reds so well. The shade of red is actually the one that the girls who dance the Nutcracker in Westport wear for their performances. I also lined the lips with a deep berry lipliner around the edges to give a bit of depth.

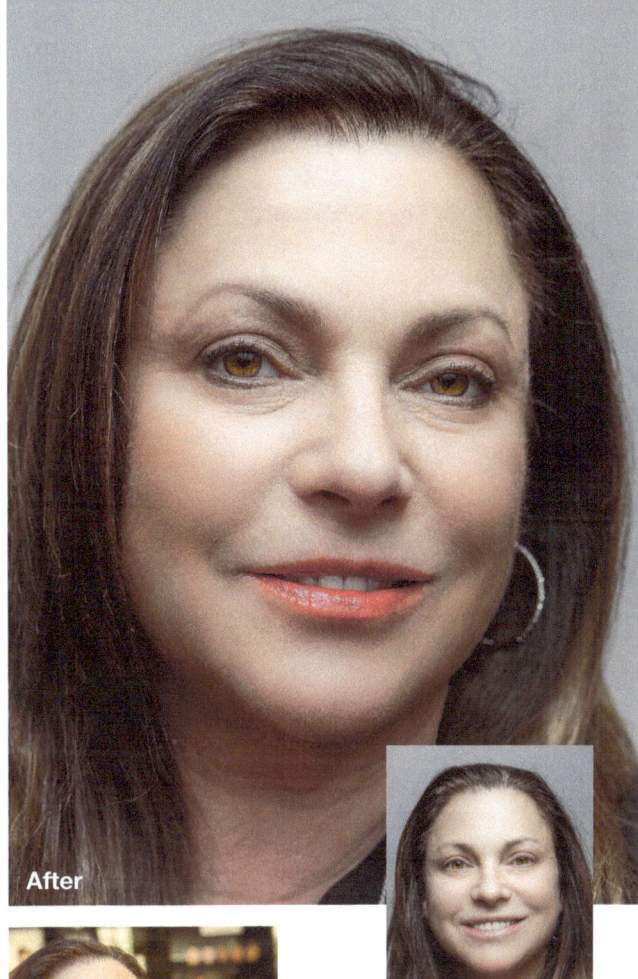

After

Before

Even without makeup, you can see Carol, at 63, has fabulous bone structure and full lips. These are exactly the features I want to focus on.

Wow! This is so good. Thank you so much for including me in your book. I am sure it will be a success. Maybe a new career for me?

Carol

How to Choose Face Makeup

The point of foundation is to help your skin look its best, not to look like you're wearing layers of makeup. The first step is finding a product that is right for your individual skin type. A tinted moisturizer or a BB cream doesn't offer as much coverage as a foundation. Choose a heavier foundation if your skin truly needs it or it's an event that warrants it. For women over 50, it's best to look for moisturizing formulas that won't settle into fine lines and wrinkles. Don't go for a powder foundation or anything with a matte finish. These types of foundations can dry out your skin and settle into fine lines and wrinkles.

One of the reasons that women love to get tan is most of us feel that darker, bronzed skin is more youthful. Remember this when you're choosing your foundation/tinted moisturizer color. Everyone has different facial skin tones. If you want a deeper tone, you should choose the darker of your shades to match. I typically like to match the tone of the décolleté, as it is typically a shade or two darker then your facial skin or the neck tone. If you choose a tone too light, it will actually accentuate fine lines and wrinkles. When you're applying your foundation, don't forget about the spot where your jaw line meets your neck. Make sure your face is blended into the top of your neck as well.

You should test the color on your face or on your jaw line. If the lighting in the store isn't bright enough, then walk outside if you want to get a better view.

A big mistake many women make is that they choose a color that blends well just with their neckline. The neck sees the least of the sunshine over our lifetimes, so it stands to reason that it's paler than your face and your décolleté. But if your décolleté is as light as your neck, then choose the light color when matching for your facial color. When I'm choosing a color for a client, I don't look at just her face. I look at her face, her neck, and her décolleté all at once and choose a color that enhances all, blends well, and is a texture that melds into the skin, rather than just sits there. Hence, this is why everyone loves my "Brush On Liquid Mineral Makeup".

It always surprises me to learn that some women only own one type of foundation and only one color. Makeup is seasonal, like clothing. In the summer months, you need a makeup product that is lighter weight, maybe with less oils, more SPF, and probably a darker shade. In the winter, I prefer a makeup product that is creamier, not a dry, matte finish. Also, don't be afraid to mix colors. I use two different foundation colors for summer and winter, depending how much sun I've gotten, and mix them together in between those two seasons.

You know dewy skin is in. It's more youthful and once you hit a certain age, it may be harder to have naturally dewy skin. I rarely use powder on more mature skin. I prefer a setting mist. Yes, sometimes in the summer or in very humid climates I will set with a powder. But, when I do apply powder, I don't do it right after I apply the makeup. I wait unit the very end of the makeup routine, so I can see how the makeup has settled. Then just before I put on the lips, I'll add a touch of powder.

Concealers Are My Least Favorite Make-Up Product

Concealing under eyes, covering shadows and dark spots are big problems for all women, and this only gets worse with age. The best way to rid under eye circles is with plenty of sleep, limit your intake of alcohol and caffeine, and use an eye cream with lightening and brightening ingredients.

"You'll never be as young as you are today."

If you must use a concealer, you already know that most of them crease, even though they promise not to. I say don't put it on first, as many makeup artists recommend. I say apply it last. It's best to apply concealer after foundation because once you cover up with a foundation, even on your bad spots, you may notice you need less concealer. I like to choose a concealer that is a slight shade darker than your skin. Remember, lighter shades tend to show more wrinkles. I don't go for that "sunglass tan line" look. I also like to mix a concealer with peach or pink tones to off set the darkness that comes through the skin. I apply concealer with a brush, as it actually places less product under the eye area. And, remember – less is more.

Should You Call the Plastic Surgeon?

Wanting to look young is not exactly a new idea -- the search for the fountain of youth has been going on for centuries. If everything that you are doing is not giving you the look that you want, there are plenty of cosmetic procedures that will.

"It's not about what happens to you in life. It's about how you deal with it..."

Dermatologists, plastic surgeons, and medi spas offer quite an array of non-invasive temporary solutions, as well as more permanent and more invasive procedures. Laugh lines can be plumped up with a wide assortment of fillers. Brow muscles can be softened with injectables derived from the botulinum toxin, best known as Botox®. For a higher price and a bit of down time, there are chemical peels, dermabrasion, laser resurfacing, light treatments, and other new cosmetic technology, all of which are effective in reducing wrinkles and discoloration. If you want more permanency, want to really smooth and lift both your face and neck, aren't opposed to spending more money, and are accepting of a longer recovery time, there are many face-lift surgical techniques. If you're considering any of these cosmetic procedures, do your homework and research it thoroughly. There's no one right answer. How you age and what steps you take to enhance your youth is entirely personal. For me, it's my home care regimen, my weekly chemical peels with my esthetician, and my bi-annual dose of Juvederm® and Botox® that keep me in check.

EYES

The Second Essential Element for Living Beautifully

It's All About the Eyes…

The idea is, as you get older, you want eyes that "look" natural, which mean they look like you haven't gone overboard with makeup. And while looking natural can take a bit of effort, it's worth a little extra time. Especially for your daily look, you don't want to appear as if you're wearing a lot of makeup.

> **"Appreciate where you are in life today.**
> **Tomorrow you'll be older."**

I'm going to introduce you to two must know techniques. Start with an eye shadow primer to keep eye shadow in place all day, especially if you're using a light color. Drooping eyelids are a normal part of aging women, so let's just learn the eye shadow techniques that make you look your best. You can spend thousands on an eyelift, or you can try my beauty tips that cost nothing to conceal your crepe-y lids. Use a light hand. You can always apply extra coats. In this book, these are the only two eye shadow techniques applied. On each woman, I will share which technique I used and which colors I actually applied to achieve her look. Both techniques are simple to follow and only require two or three eye shadow colors. You can refer back to this page for any one of the women as a reminder to the steps for each of my eye shadow techniques.

Many makeup artists suggest keeping eyeliner to the upper lid only. I am a rule-breaker makeup artist, so I think you can go ahead and line the bottom lashes with a gel or soft pencil and smudge it with a smudge brush, a sponge, or your finger. Be sure to set it with a little eye shadow to keep it in place. I also like to layer in eyeliners. I may start with a gel or kohl pencil for the top liner, apply the eye shadow and then come back and apply a liquid liner to add a crisp, enhanced look. It all depends on the look I'm going for and the lasting power I'm trying to achieve. Sometimes I'll curve the line up on the outer corners of eyes to lift them. But definitely avoid thick, heavy lines, whether on the top or bottom.

Shimmer eye shadows, sparkle eye shadows, frosted eye shadows, glitter eye shadows, satin eye shadows, sheen eye shadows – what are these? All of these describe eye shadows with an assortment of small light reflective particles. The shadows that have large particles can be your worst enemy, because heavy shimmer eye shadows only highlight crow's feet and make eyes look even more crepe-y. Shadows that have very finely ground particles such as satin and sheen eye shadows can actually reflect the light in such as way as it is deflecting your fine lines and highlighting your eyes in a very helpful way. One area where satin and sheen finishes work in is the area just over your pupil to make your eyes pop.

The Reverse Nude Eye Shadow Technique

Do you ever hear about women that complain that they have no eyelid, or they're trying to make their eyelid very light, thinking it will help to make their eyelid pop more? If you have lids that aren't clearly visible when your eye is open, then the Reverse Nude Eye Shadow Technique is one that you should absolutely know.

You can do this in three easy steps, using only three colors. The three steps are: one color for your lid, one color to blend into your contour, and then eyeliner.

Step 1: LID – Using a flat eye shadow brush, slightly damp with water, apply a medium to dark shade of eye shadow over your entire lid. Starting from the lash line, apply with a pressing motion from the lash line to the contour bone area, or slightly above.

Step 2: CONTOUR – Using a lighter shade of eye shadow take a large blending brush, place the color at your contour area of your eye, and blend in towards your nose. Blend over the contour, into the highlight area, but not all the way to your brow line. This technique doesn't require you to highlight your brow area—that's optional.

Step 3: LINER – You can use a small angled eyeliner brush or a small smudge brush slightly wet with water. Dip into the darkest shade of the trio of eye shadows you've selected. Apply the shadow liner to both the top and bottom lash lines in a wiggle motion. Do not try to draw a line. Lots of little wiggles and dashes will ultimately form a straight line with your lash line.

Optional eyeliner technique: Gel Liner – You could also line with a gel pencil instead of an eye shadow or in addition to your eye shadow liner. Starting at the outer corner of your lash line, apply the gel pencil with small dashes, pushing into your lash line. You can use your smudge brush or angle brush to blend. Using this technique along the top lash line creates a fuller lash appearance.

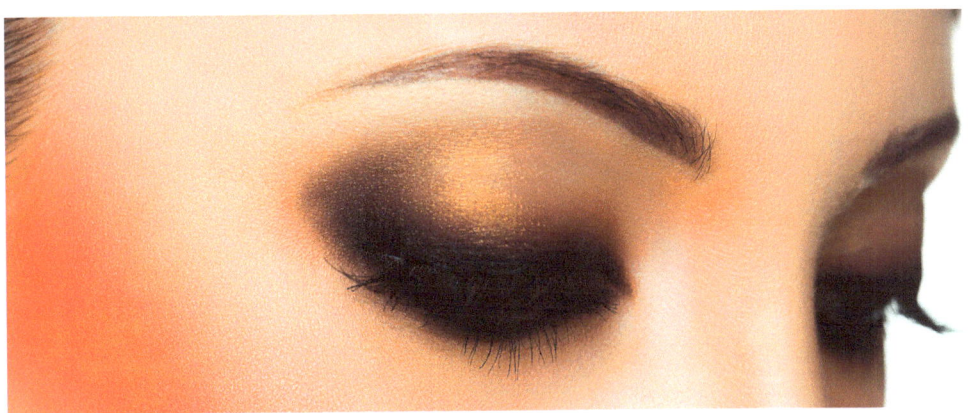

19

The Side "V" Eye Shadow Technique

The Side "V" Eye Shadow Technique is essentially a spin off on the Classic Nude Eye Shadow Technique, which I taught in my last book. What the Side "V" does better is that it doesn't place a deeper color into the entire contour, which would make the face look more angular and therefore older. This is exactly what we want to avoid. The Side "V" Technique is more youthful, as the side-ways "V" at the edge of the eye creates an uplifting look.

You can do this in three easy steps, using only three colors. The three steps are: one color for your lid, one color to blend into your V-contour, and then eyeliner. You can use the same colors for your Side "V" as you used for you Reverse Nude, you're just going to swap the placement of the colors. In a Side "V", the lightest color goes on the lid, whereas in a Reverse Nude, the darkest color goes on the lid.

Step 1: LINE – Start by lining your eyes, choosing the darkest shadow from your trio of colors. You can use a wet shadow as a liner, or a pencil. Apply the liner to the upper and lower lashes, smudging them a bit so they don't have a harsh line. Pull the line up just a bit at the outside corner.

Step 2: LID – Selecting the lightest of the color trio you've chosen, use a light touch to sweep the color over the lid from the lash line to the crease area.

Optional POP – To further accentuate your eyes, you can add a highlighter right in the center of the eyelid, over your pupil. You would choose a color similar or lighter to the color on your lid. This shadow will have a sheen finish and it is that sheen that will give your eyes a special pop. You can extend the highlighter over your lids to the inside corner of the eyes.

Step 3: "V"- Choose a color darker than the lid color for this step. Using a brush that places color, create a side-ways "V"-shape in which the open part of the "V" faces in towards the nose. After you've created your "V" shape, blend it in towards the nose with a blending brush from the outside of the eye going in towards the lid.

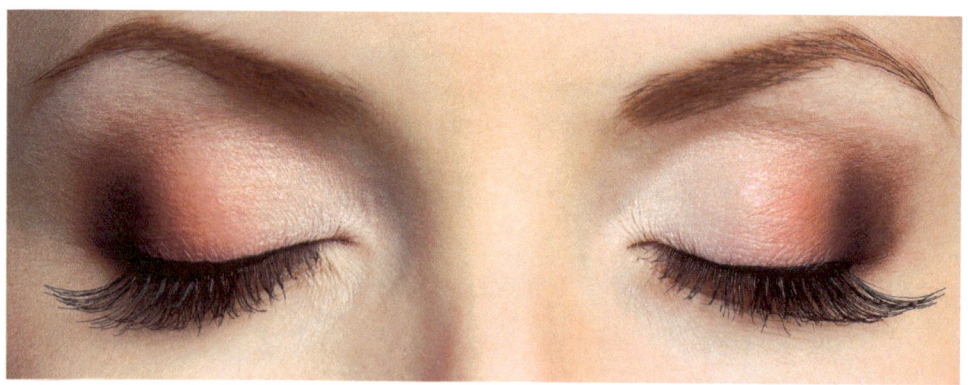

Lindsey's natural transformation

I started with a primer to give her skin extra smoothness. Then I applied our liquid mineral makeup and as I was blending, I added a touch of the mineral tinted moisturizer to give a more luminous and creamy glow.

For her eyes, I used neutral shades of shadows with the **Reverse Nude Eye Shadow Technique**. After this, I applied gel eyeliners

- **LID** – Apply a dark taupe eye shadow to the eye lid
- **CONTOUR** – Contour the eyelid using a medium taupe eye shadow
- **LINER** – Apply black liner on the top and bottom
- **GEL LINER** – Use a black gel liner on the top, and a deep blue liner in the inner water line on the bottom.
- **MASCARA** – Apply a very black mascara to top and bottom lashes.

For Lindsey's cheeks, using my **Bronze & Blush Face Lift Technique**. I choose a warm shade of bronzer for under her cheekbones. I also applied it over her eyebrows and into her hairline, as well as under her chin, along her jawline, and over her neck area. Then I finished the look with a touch of pink blush just above the bronzer on her cheekbones. I added concealer under her eyes at the end. I find applying the concealer last, lets me use less then when I apply it at the very beginning.

More glow - With my fingers, I put a highlighter with across her cheeks, under her eyes and at the top of her eye shadow into her forehead.

For her lips, Lindsey prefers gloss and pale colors. So, I mixed a pale, cool violet lipstick, which really pops her blue eyes with a shinny nude gloss.

The look was natural – Not naked!

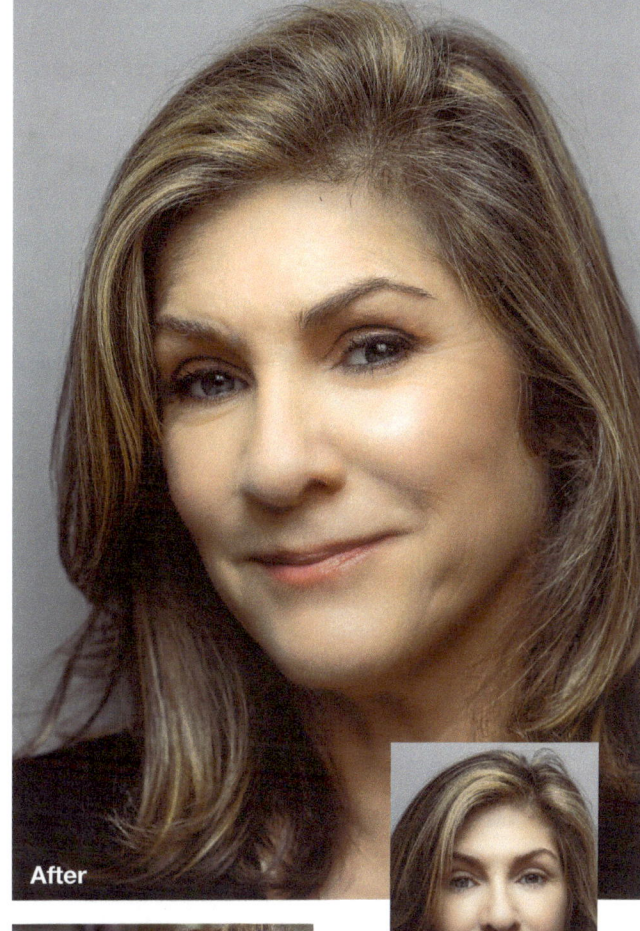

After

Before

Lindsey, who looks a lot like Jennifer Aniston, is a no makeup kind of makeup girl. She likes to look fresh and natural. But we all know at our age natural certainly doesn't mean naked. It means the perfect balance of getting enough makeup on without looking like you tried too hard.

For her look, I want to highlight Lindsey's exceptional eyebrows, which already frame her pretty blue eyes beautifully. Let's see how I can enhance that frame…

> *Loved last night! Seeing the results of your magic is always fantastic! The atmosphere was great. Being with women who are all in the same age group and the vibe that you always bring to the party just makes it fun!*
>
> *Lindsey*

Next, use an eyelash curler. Curling your lashes can do wonders to open up your eyes at every age. My little secret… I warm up my eyelash curler with a shot of the blow dryer for about three seconds, before curling my lashes.

Eye pencils come in many different textures and firmness. I recommend the ones that are soft, either gel or kohl pencils. These lend themselves to smudging easily, which is what you want. Also, most women don't realize that once you apply a pencil, smudge it to achieve the look you want, it then should be layered with a similar color eye shadow to "set" it into place. This is an especially important technique if you live in very warm or humid climates. Or, if you have those types of eyes that with each blink you hit the tops and bottoms of your eyelid and are constantly smudging your makeup, then "setting" is a must.

Learn the Lush Lash Trick – No More Clumpy Eye Lashes!

Eyelashes thin over time. That's just a side effect of this aging process. But you can fight it. You can try mascaras that have thickeners in them, absolutely thoroughly remove your mascara every night, replace your mascara every three months, and apply nightly one of the many lash boosting serums, which are filled with vitamins and moisturizers to enhance lashes. If you don't have good lashes you might consider getting eyelash extensions or individual false lashes. Also, decide that its time to master the eyeliner techniques that I'm sharing in these two techniques.

> **"Women tell me they want to look natural. But, natural doesn't mean naked. Girls, get enough makeup on so you can 'look' natural."**

Start by applying mascara with the wand from the base of your eyelashes. Do not re-dip the wand, but instead rotate it to use up the mascara on all sides. Then hold the wand in a vertical position and begin to separate the lashes and pull out to the sides, a bit like a wing effect. Curl upper lashes after the first coat. Think about when you apply hair product to your hair. Your hair styles the best when there is already product in your hair for pliability. The same is true with your eyelashes. You can really make them thick and get them to wing out after the first coat and after curling. The second coat and the vertical application really makes your lashes pop. Look at the pictures of Rivers and Lindsey to see how I hold the wand and separate their lashes.

Be careful when applying mascara to your bottom lashes. Go lightly and use the vertical application technique. Just a little is all you are looking for. Also, don't start at the center. The first few strokes should be at the outside corners.

EYEBROWS Are Queen

Eyebrows count! You know why? Your eyebrows literally frame your eyes. It's all about your eyes. I'm affectionately known as the Eyebrow Queen. Most women say my brow shaping is almost like getting a mini facelift. A good shape can really lift your face. The frame has to compliment the picture. If they're not shaped right or filled in, then you're just not going to look as great as you could. Your eyebrows, or lack thereof, could be adding years to your face. After all, they are your most defining feature, and now that they're sparser—maybe even coarser and grayer—they're not doing your face any favors.

Our eyebrows are expressive as they tell others when we're surprised, happy, sad, or concerned. But, if they are poorly shaped or too thin, the only thing they'll show is your age. I feel that full, well-shaped brows are the most essential attribute to an overall youthful look. They open and highlight your eyes, making you look alert and sparkling.

Sadly, eyebrows do thin out over the years. Thinner eyebrows have a variety of causes, ranging from over plucking, over waxing, menopause, taking certain medications to sleeping on the same side of your pillow. Over time, brows naturally thin at the outer edges, by your temples. The tail of the brow is the part that makes the arch; it's the sexy part of the brow. Because, it's all about the eyes.

How to Enhance Your Eyebrows:

See an eyebrow expert for shaping. Most cities and towns, no matter how small, have someone or someplace that specializes in eyebrow shaping. Don't try to shape your own eyebrows. It's a bit like cutting your own hair – hard to do on yourself. One of the reasons that doing your own brows is so difficult is that we are all asymmetrical people and your right side will never match your left side.

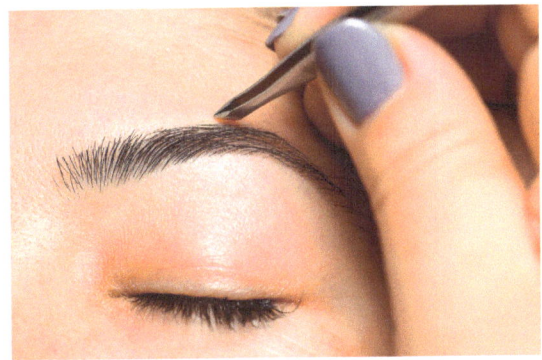

Here are some of my eyebrow shaping tricks. I hope you'll share them with your eyebrow artist, but I'm sure that some of you will master these on your own.

Brows need to be tweezed from the top too! If you only pluck from the bottom, your brows will probably appear too high. Shaping at the top helps to create the arch.

I strongly suggest shaping eyebrows while you are seated in an upright position, not lying down. I know a lot of brow people like to wax brows while you are lying down. First of all, I am not a fan of waxing, especially for women who are 40+, because waxing pulls at your skin and weakens the collagen, which is the very thing you need to keep your skin tight and firm. I'm also not a believer in lying down while shaping brows, regardless of what type of hair remover your brow specialist is using. When you lie down your face lies down too. Your skin relaxes when you're lying down. What's important to me is how your eyebrows look when others are looking at you, which is how your skin looks in its natural state. If one brow has a natural position, which causes it to sit lower, then your other brow, this can be adjusted during the brow shaping.

One important concern is if you want to have an arch, then how do you determine where the arch should go? The trick here is to open your eyes and the top of the arch should be aligned with the outside of your pupil or your iris. The actual location depends on your eye size. Be here's what's important. The arch should not have its height at the inside of your pupil or your iris. Many times I see women who have an arch that begins close to their nose and rises quickly before their pupil. This tends to make women look mad or makes their eyes look too close together. One of the major advantages to creating an arch, which has its height at your pupil, is that it gives your face a lift and separates your eyebrows, which in turn makes your cheekbones look higher.

I have a few more suggestions for you. I definitely recommend filling in sparse brows. This is one of my daily regiment. I cannot go anywhere without my brows. You'll never see me au natural. There are so many good brow fillers to choose from. Try a few and see what you like best. Choose from: brow powder, brow balm, brow liners, brow pencils, and brow gels. You should consider the amount of humidity where you live, the moisture of your skin, and the longevity of different products.

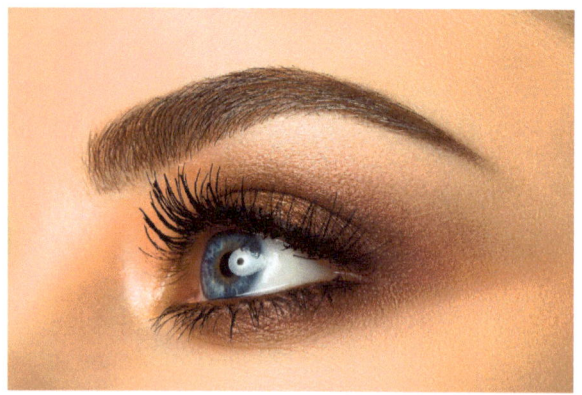

I also love tinting eyebrows. It's not the same as filling them. But, if you have enough brow hair and you just want to cover greys or to give a great contrast of color, then tint them. And, if you are in need of growing more eyebrows, then you should try one of the many brow serums, which stimulate hair growth. By the way, most of the products on the market, which stimulate eyelash growth, also stimulate eyebrow growth. The key is to use the product daily. By the way, the picture on the left shows a woman wearing the Reverse Nude Eye Shadow Technique.

Eyebrows Are Unique and Individual to Each Woman

One brow does not fit all.

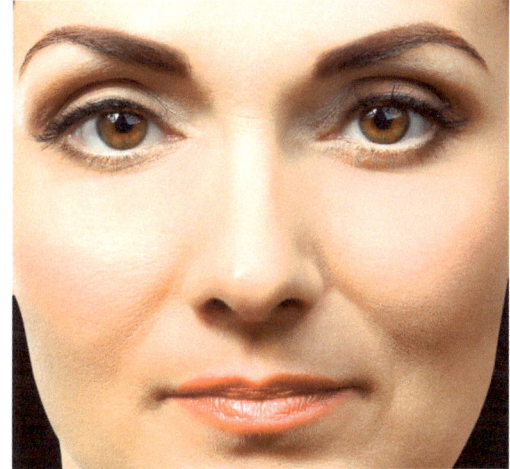

Perfect wide-set eyebrow arches. This woman is also wearing the Side "V" Eye Shadow Technique with a POP.

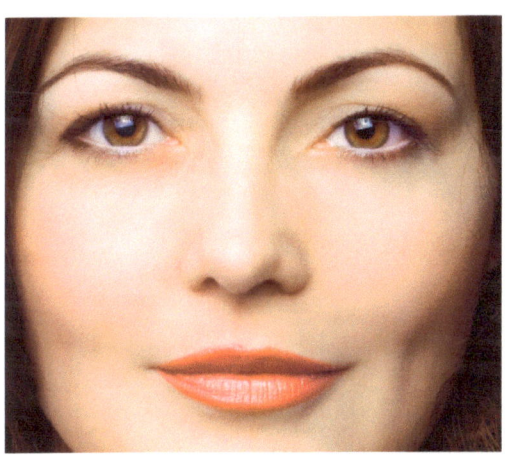

Oval-shaped eyebrows don't have a pinnacle arched peak. Especially good for square-shaped faces. This woman is also wearing the Side "V" Eye Shadow Technique.

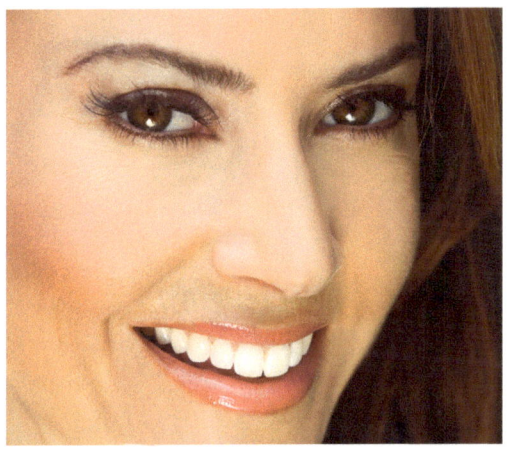

Some eyebrows need wispy hairs. Imagine how awkwardly wide the space above her nose would be without those hairs. She is wearing the Reverse Nude Eyeshadow Technique.

Tami

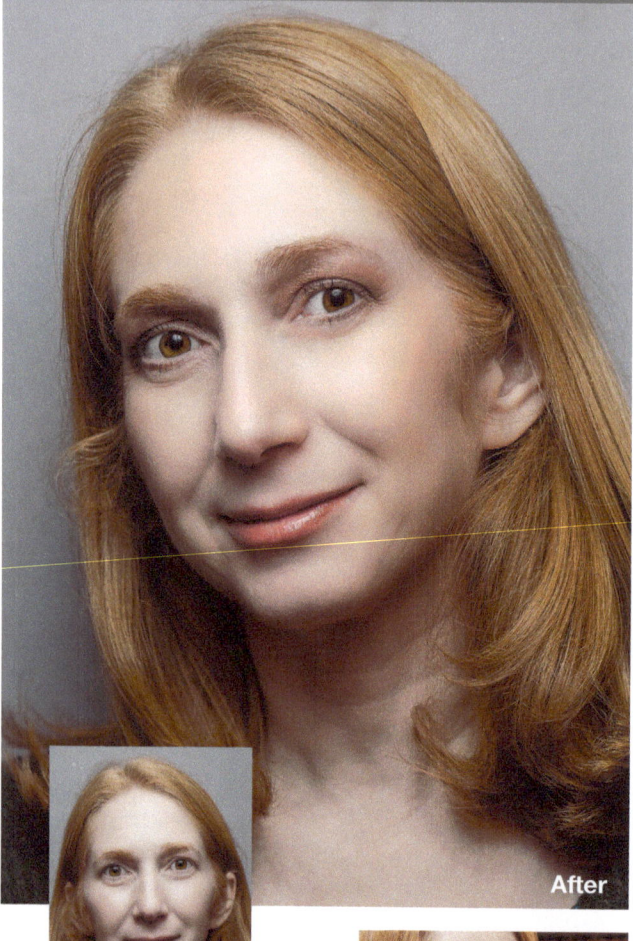

Reds can go with fall colors...

I started with a hydrating toner, followed with a primer. And, then I applied a liquid mineral makeup on Tami's face. I choose this shade of foundation to warm up her overall skin tones.

For Tami's eyebrows, I wanted a softer look. I began by using a slightly moist brush and I dipped it into a shade of eye shadow that most closely matched Tami's eyebrows. I filled in her brows just a bit more on the ends.

For her eyes, I used my **Side "V" Eye Shadow Technique**.

- **LINE** – Apply brown eyeliner on top and bottom
- **LID** – Apply amber and beige eye shadows
- **"V"** – Apply a cognac shade of eye shadow in the "V"
- **POP** – Mix a white and a beige eye shadow to pop the eye
- **MASCARA** – Apply black mascara to top and bottom lashes.

For Tami's cheeks, I used my **Bronze & Blush Face Lift Technique**. I applied a warm shade of bronzer over her eyebrows, added a touch into her hairline, and added just a bit over her nose. Then I followed with just a touch of coral blush, above the bronzer at the very top of her cheekbones by her hairline.

I wanted a natural look with a hint of a warm apricot tone for Tami's lips. I filled them in with a spice colored lip liner and used a pale coral gloss over it for a very natural, yet long wearing natural look.

After

Before

Tami is a beautiful 46-year-old redhead. One choice as a red head is to do a monochromatic look. When I did a monochromatic look on Rivers on page 27, who is blonde, I choose blonde-type pale, neutral colors. For Tami, I chose warm ambers, oranges, browns, and cognac shades. I want to bring the warmth of Tami's hair and spread that glow of sunshine all over her face.

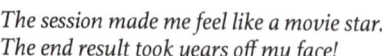

The session made me feel like a movie star. The end result took years off my face!

Tami

What to Do in a Beauty Rush?

When you find yourself in a beauty rush with only minutes to apply makeup, I recommend applying any two of these:

• Tinted moisturizer/foundation
• Mascara
• Blush
• Lipstick
• Eyebrows

Pick two and that's all you really need to look flawless.

> **"Lips are made for kissing, so make them gorgeous!"**

Young Youthful LIPS

I despise those vertical lines above my mouth! They call them smoker's lines! Not fair. I don't even smoke. They look just awful and nothing makes you look older, faster. I hear so much about lip fillers like Juvederm® and Restylane®. There are lots of women who do fillers in the lip area and look great. But I'm afraid that I'll look all puffy mouthed and "fish-faced". I tend to remember the ones that are over exaggerated and fear that's how they will come out on me. Also, once you start with lip filler, it's addicting. If you stop, the lines may look a lot worse. So, is there another answer to aging, thinning lips and those wrinkled lines that form around our mouths?

The first tip in helping the lips look full is exfoliation. As we age, our lips lose their natural oils and their plumpness. To maintain your full plump factor and keep lips looking smooth, make sure to keep your lips exfoliated all year round. I could give you a list of homemade remedies of lip scrubs or products on the market, but the truth is we all hate to have to take even one more step in our routine, so I'll make it easy for you. All it takes is brushing your lips with your toothbrush. Every time you brush your teeth, brush your lips too. And then add a touch of lip balm, your lip-gloss, or a hydrating lipstick.

Go Lipstick Shopping

Lipstick shopping is just like shopping for a pair of eyeglasses. You have to try lots on and pare it down to just a few. Don't go lipstick shopping without any makeup on. Put on your normal face, or if a nighttime lip is what you're looking for, try lip colors with your night makeup. I'm not a big fan of the color doctrine predetermining the colors that are right for which skin tones. I feel like those rules that say blondes should always do this or light skin women are often too limiting. You should experiment with colors.

Do You Dare Wear Bright and Bold Lips?

Bright lipstick is especially stunning on women who wear glasses. The bold lip balances out the heaviness of the frames. Just remember to balance your eye makeup and blush if you are going bold on your lips. Many of us want to have a full youthful pout. While lighter shades tend to make lips look bigger and poutier than darker shades, that doesn't mean you can't wear darker shades. A too-pale shade can make you look as if you are wearing no lipstick at all. If this is what you're going after, great, but most of us want a little pop of color. If you have thin lips, keep in mind that super dark colors may make your lips look like they have disappeared into your mouth leaving two thin lines. There are many bright, bold lip colors that can be flattering.

> **"Try something new. Show me a person who has never made a mistake and I'll show you a person who has never lived."**

Lip Liner Makes Fuller Lips

Here's how not to wear lip liner - Never draw an exact dark line around the edge of your lips and just leave the obvious dark line there. To make your lips appear larger with liner, start by applying your lipstick, with a brush to your natural lip line. The trick is after the lipstick is applied, then using a similar shade of liner, draw the lip liner just outside your natural lip line, which you can easily see with the lip color applied, right above the bow of your top lip and just outside the fattest part of your lower lip. Don't line the corners on the outside of the natural line. Fill in the rest of the lips with the lipstick and top with a touch of gloss on the pouty part of the bottom lip. By the way, if you fill your entire lip first with a lip liner it will double as a lip stain and give you longer-lasting color. Of course, you can always apply a long-lasting lipstick or stain on top.

Bronze & Blush Face Lift Technique

This technique frames your eyes and perks your cheeks. Overall it gives the illusion of a more open and lifted look.

1. Using a flat topped face brush, apply your bronzer in a triangular shape under the cheekbone. Start at the outer edge of your face, by your hairline and ear.

2. Without redipping your bronzer brush, bronze the area on your forehead, above your eyes, into your hairline.

3. Using a round top or dome topped face brush, apply your blush just higher than your bronzer and blend into your bronzer. Begin blush at the top of your cheek, closest to your hairline. Do not start at your apple area. That area will have less color than the outside to of your cheek.

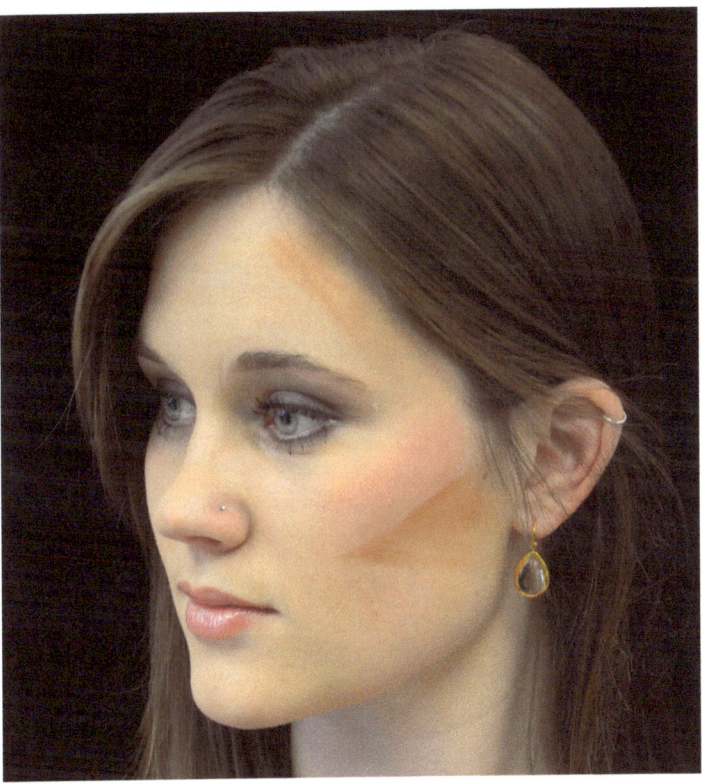

"Bronzer and blush applied properly are like a good underwire bra – they lift you right up!"

Do You Need Bronzer or Blush?

One beauty trick I love is how bronzer highlights your eyes and gives you a little lift. Bronzer, when applied under your cheekbone area and applied in an opposing angle by your hairline, highlights your eyes and gives your cheeks a lift.

Bronzer can also add dimension to your face. This technique is known as contouring. It's a technique that can be useful for creating a lift. I say it does for our cheeks what a good underwire bra does for our "girls". Bronzers and blush create definition to the face. The goal here is to create shadows to highlight your best parts, hello cheekbones, and downplay an older chin or turkey neck. Applied along the jawline, on the temples and under the chin, bronzer can give your face a more angled, leaner look.

Choose Bronzer and a Blush

Most everyone feels slimmer, sexier, and prettier with a tan. A bronzer can also have that effect on you, adding color to an otherwise sallow face. Too many women use blush incorrectly or not at all. A pop of blush on the apples of your cheeks can brighten a dull complexion. But the trick is to blend it well so it's not obvious you're wearing blush. I see too many women who look as if they've painted the blush on their faces in the dark, which brings me to my next tip.

In my book, *Making Faces Beautiful*, I spent a great deal of time drawing the angles on top of the faces of the models. I did this so you could see the angles that I was going to apply to each woman's face in order to accentuate or further enhance her features. You can check out that book, if you want to get the full demonstration. But for this group of women, I'm going to focus on how to highlight each woman's eyes. I do that first with either my Reverse Nude Eye Shadow Technique and my Side "V" Shadow Technique.

Under the eye, lies the cheeks and cheekbone. Over the eye is the forehead and the hairline. When bronzer and blush are applied using my Bronze & Blush Face Lift Technique, it's as if you've gotten a real lift.

"Bronzer and blush should lift and separate. Hmm... I wonder where I heard that?"

Are Highlighters Helpful?

After all of this conversation on choosing the darker of your skin tones, bronzed skin makes your look leaner and younger. Why would anyone want to use a highlighter, which makes them look lighter? It's just another one of those beauty tricks that when used properly, the lightness with a touch of sheen, next to the darker, more matte skin gives a more refreshed, lifted, and awake appearance. I like to use the pads of my fingers and swipe the highlighter over the darker areas of the face: at the tops of the cheeks, under the outsides of the eyes, by corners of the mouth, and by the sides of the nose.

Rivers' blonde monochromatic look...

First I hydrated and plumped Rivers' skin with a hydrating toner and moisture cream. To get that gorgeous glow that you see on Rivers, I mixed about a quarter size of tinted moisturizer with a tiny dash of cream highlighter and applied the mixture to her face and neck using my fingers and a foundation brush. Wow, that skin! For daytime she could do this look too—just throw on a pair of big sunglasses, apply a bright lipstick, and go!

Continuing on to brows and eyes-- Rivers has good brows to follow. However, they still needed some filling in. For her eyes I chose shades of pale pinks using the **Side "V" Eye Shadow Technique** and extra layers of a gel eye liner.

- **LINE** – Apply a black eyeliner on top and bottom
- **LID** – Mix a light pink and a white eye shadow
- **"V"** – Apply a rose shade of eye shadow in the "V"
- **POP** – Apply a light pink eye shadow with sheen
- **GEL LINER** – Use a black gel eye liner
- **MASCARA** – Apply a black mascara to top and bottom lashes.

To pop her cheeks I did my tried and true **Bronze & Blush Face Lift Technique**. I also applied the bronzer over her eyes, under her chin, jaw, and neck area. Then I applied a coral blush just at and above her cheek area.

For her lips, I choose a medium coral/pink lipstick because Rivers has a great mouth and loves lipstick. I then lined her lips with a touch of a berry liner and glossed them over with just a touch of a pale neutral gloss.

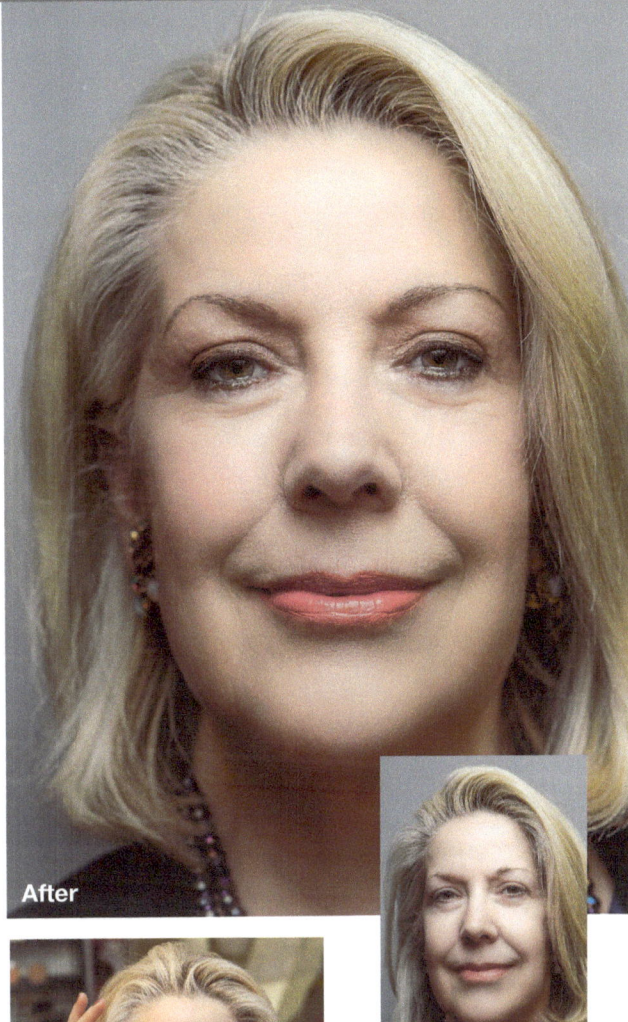

After

Before

Rivers is a fair-skinned maiden. She is serene, calm, and lovely. I wanted to give her a look that reflected her inner self, so I choose to go with a soft monochromatic look. I know this is not Rivers' norm, as she typically dresses in strong cool colors and her makeup balances with those bright pinks, greens, and blues. But, I'm going with soft pinks, soft corals, and neutral tones because I think will make her blonde hair and blue eyes really come alive.

Thank you so much for inviting me to participate in your glamorous night of makeovers. I loved the way you did my makeup and now the new lip colors I am going to have for the winter. I came home and studied all the details in my mirror in trying to replicate those eyes!

Rivers

Does Your Style Accentuate Your Eyes?

What does your style say about you? I want my style to say I'm happy, confident, healthy, and did you notice my big green eyes? Your style is the picture that people see first. You're spending all of this time making your skin glow and focusing on make up techniques, which is all very important. But I want you to give an extra thought to hairstyling and what clothing you wear.

I think that women, especially women who are 50+ should choose clothes that are comfortable, but stylish. That doesn't mean dressing like a teenager. I think many women in America are so hung up on comfort that they walk around in sweat clothes all day. Unless you are running errands from yoga class, in Lululemon – which makes everyone's butt look great, don't do it. You can have so much fun with fashion. You just need to find the formula that fits your body shape, your age, and lifestyle.

And, don't get stuck on numbers. Bodies change and every clothing manufacturer sizes differently. Many women shop by size only and get stuck on the idea that if they are an 8 in one company that they're always an 8, even when they might be a 10 or a 12 in another manufacturer. Buy clothes that fit, not the number you want to be and your clothes will look so much better.

Be fashionable, not trendy. Not every look works for every person. I prefer classic looks and classic colors. My wardrobe includes lots of basic pieces in a few neutral colors. Basic and classic pieces can still be edgy. Just keep it well-tailored or have a unique trim to a classic piece. Be basic, but not boring. Buy some timeless garments, such as sleek black pants or button up white shirts that you can mix and match for a classic look. I choose slender pants, longer sweaters, and always love dresses. When I choose an outfit, I always start with the shoe that I want to wear. Your wardrobe needs an assortment of comfortable, stylish flats and boots, as well as wearable, stylish heels and boots. When you have happy feet, the rest is easy.

> ## "It's not about what size you wear, it's how you wear your size."

Now that your wardrobe is classic and stylish, you can embellish with your hair, makeup, and accessories. That's right, your hair and makeup are accessories too. An up to date hairstyle can take years off of you. The right hairstyle and hair color can take years off of you. Talk to your hairstylist, talk to a new stylist, do your research, but if you're' wearing the same cut and color that you were wearing a decade ago, there's a good chance your look is expired.

Accessorize to spice up your classic clothing. As a mature dresser, stock your wardrobe with attention-getting pieces. Purchase a few scarves, interesting earrings, an arm of bangles, a few fabulous necklaces, a coordinating belt, and you always need great handbags and stunning shoes. With the addition of these accessories, you can give every outfit style. And, here's a secret that took us 50+ years to learn: You're more comfortable in your skin than you've ever been, so wear it with style.

Pam

The balancing act

Pam's skin is so cool-based. I wanted to add a little warmth to her skin. I did so by blending a tinted moisturizer with a touch of a cream concealer. The concealer provided a little more coverage and the tone of it also added some warmth.

I filled Pam's eyebrows with a slightly damp small angle eye shadow brush and I applied a tiny bit of black eye shadow and lightly stroked it over her natural brow lines.

As you can see from the picture, Pam is holding my lucite palette that has all of my colors in it. I put together eggplant and brown eye shadows, using the **Reverse Nude Eye Shadow Technique**.

- **LID** – Apply brown eye shadow to the eyelids
- **CONTOUR** – Apply an eggplant colored eye shadow to contour the eyelid
- **LINER** – Apply black eyeliner on top, and brown eyeliner on bottom
- **GEL LINER** – Apply black liner on the top
- **MASCARA** – Apply mascara to top and bottom lashes.

To highlight her cheeks I applied my **Bronze & Blush Face Lift Technique**. I applied a cool-toned bronzer under her cheekbones, over her forehead, and over her neck area. Then I blended a pink gel blush just at and above her cheek area. The trick here is to smile. Before I applied her blush, I asked Pam to smile for me, and I located the apple of her cheek. I then applied the blush just a bit above her apple. If I had applied it to where I thought it was, the blush would have appeared too low and made her cheeks look droopy. This apply above the apple placement always gives the face a lift.

For her lips, I used berry colors because Pam always wears a berry colored lip well. It coordinates perfectly with her fair skin tone and her dark hair. I followed the lipstick with a deep berry lip liner and a berry gloss.

After

Before

Pam, stunning at 53, has an amazing head of dark, luxurious curly hair. However, her hair can be over powering to her face if it is not balanced out properly. She once had unruly eyebrows, which we have since tamed and shaped beautifully to her face. As full as they are, her brows actually look even better filled in. Highlighting her brows and her cheeks are the most important tricks to balancing Pam's look.

What a treat it was to be part of the "FACE it you're fabulous at every age event". Having a makeover is like hitting the reset button. It has a way of transforming you and reminding you that we ARE beautiful at any age. Gail, you are a true artist and see things in our faces that we don't. You choose colors for me I never would have on my own and I TOTALLY loved the result. I may or may not have slept with my make up on to enjoy a second day with the make up. The whole event reminded me to take the time to take care of myself. Thank you, Gail for including me in a wonderful evening.

Pam

EXERCISE

The Third Essential Element for Living Beautifully

Exercise Away Your Wrinkles...

Did you know that your facial skin, especially aging facial skin, will look more beautiful and radiant from working up a healthy sweat? Working out not only helps your figure, it also improves your complexion. Exercise is one of the best skin remedies for wrinkles and dull skin.

Whether you going on a vacation and need to trim a few pounds or are focused on staying healthy, think of all of your reasons that do include exercise in your daily routine. No matter what your motivation is, we can all agree that the benefits of exercise are good for our mind, our body, and our skin tone.

> ## "Be in control, but don't stress over what you can't control."

When you exercise, your heart rate increases and circulates more blood and oxygen to the skin. Drawing blood to the surface of the body conveys nutrients to your skin cells and helps remove toxins from the skin. When your heart gets pumping from exercise, you're supplying your skin with a nice dose of oxygenated blood, which gives you an instant youthful glow. Remember Reese Witherspoon in the movie "*Legally Blonde*"? She said exercise releases endorphins, which are feel-good chemicals that make you happier and more relaxed. When you are relaxed and happy, you look better and feel better. A more relaxed state eases lines in your skin and lowers your hormone levels.

Working out helps decrease levels of the stress-related hormone called cortisol. Too much cortisol can cause the collagen in the skin to break down, which can increase wrinkles and sagging. Collagen, which literally holds your skin together, diminishes as we age. Exercise promotes collagen in skin cells, which makes your skin age more slowly. Regular exercise boosts circulation, which in turn supports the production of collagen. As we age, the collagen producing cells in our skin diminish. It's the nutrients delivered to your skin during exercise that help the collagen producing cells to work more efficiently, so your skin looks younger. When you exercise, the tiny arteries in your skin open up, allowing more blood to reach the skin's surface and deliver nutrients that repair damage from the sun and environmental pollutants.

I offer one word of caution about excessive cardio training. Cardio is typically the exercise of choice for losing weight. Just be careful of too much running. Too much running can actually cause your face to lose its youthful elasticity. The stress placed on your body when you're running long distances produces excessive amounts of cortisol, a stress hormone responsible of creating inflammation. Between the cortisol and the sun exposure they both work at breaking down your skin's collagen, giving way to wrinkles and sagging skin. Make sure that your choice of exercises are balanced.

Quickly go from day to night

I began by blending a little liquid makeup to Ellie's face in a shade just a little deeper then what she was wearing because I wanted to deepen Ellie's overall color. I chose one deeper in tone to darken her overall skin color. I matched her décolleté, rather than matching her neck. I also applied concealer under her eye area to darken it and conceal, using a color that was also a little darker.

I then moved onto Ellie's eyebrows, filling them in using a wet angle brush with a touch of cognac color eye shadow. For her eyes, I went over her existing colors, using the plums and the rose shadows. Ellie was already doing **the Side "V" Technique**.

I started by going over her top eyeliner using a black liquid pen eyeliner. I recreated a very dramatic top line for her. I was sure to fill in the little white space that sits right at the lash line. For the under liner, I applied a dark blue eye liner pencil and set it with a dark plum eye shadow. All of this to really works to accentuate her incredible teal-colored eyes.

For her face, I did the **Bronze & Blush Face Lift Technique** in a very vertical angle as you can see from the picture.

I completed her look with an electric pink on her lips. Now, that's a very hot nighttime look. You go Ellie!!

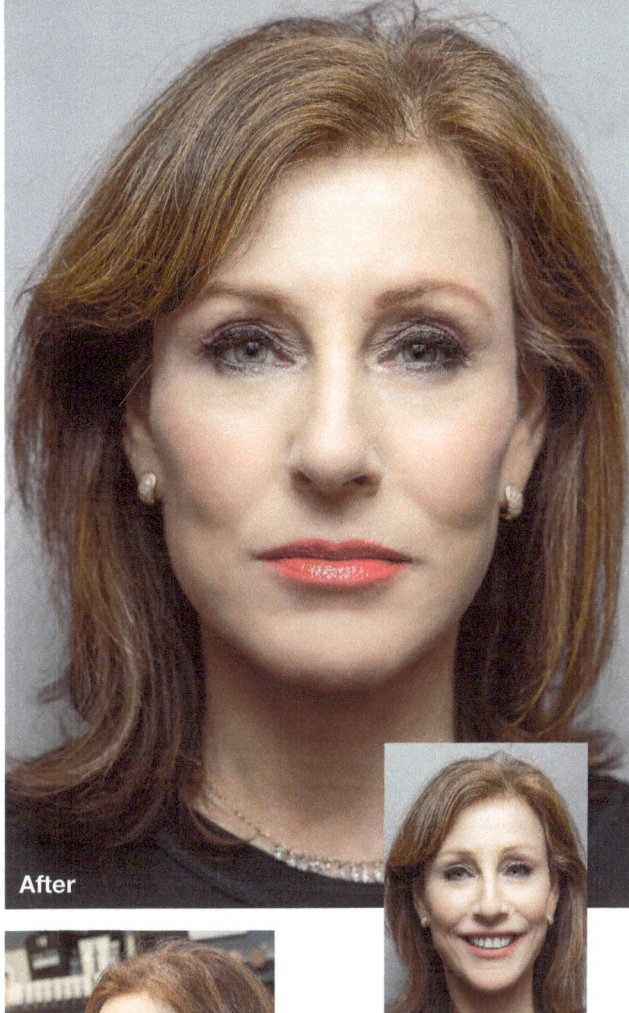

After

Before

Ellie, sexy and 63, is a very expressive and charismatic redhead. Her choice of clothing and makeup match her personality. When she came to our makeover party, she had her look on from her day. I wanted to do her makeup the same way that she already applies it, just change up the colors and show her how to turn up the volume on the techniques she already knows. I am a big fan of purples, plums, and reds for redheads.

Last night was a blast and the best part was our mutual acknowledgement of the fact that we are sisters and goddesses! Makeup only helped shine the light. You are so generous in so many ways, Gail.

Ellie

Sweating is actually healthy for you. It reduces inflammation and cleans out the pores of congested skin. This will help draw toxins out of the body. Working out and perspiration can correct hormonal imbalances that causes

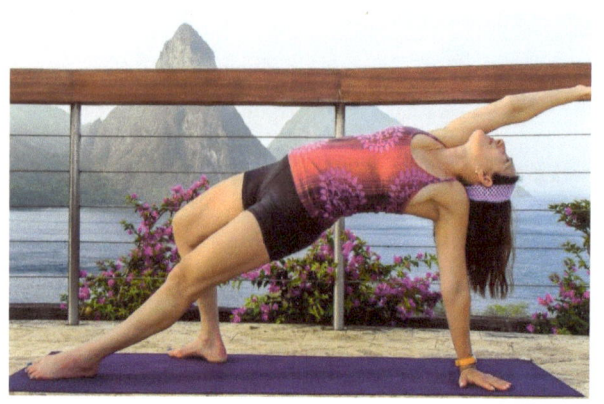

adult acne. Exercise tones your complexion, leaving your facial skin firmer, more supple and with greater elasticity. You can tone your facial skin in much the same way as you tone your muscles. As we age, our skin naturally loses its plumping, youthful layer of fat. It's the lean muscle mass that sits just under the surface which can create a lifted, taught looking, firmer facial skin.

Having youthful skin takes all five of my E's to achieve it. Every woman has her go-to village of people to offer support and advice. An important member of my village is my trainer and close friend, Lory Braun Wasserman. For over a decade Lory and I focus on the many ways it takes to look young, feel young, and stay young. We found our bond because she wanted to work on her culinary skills and I wanted to improve my workout. Lory has over dozen certifications, in everything from yoga to cycling. That's Lory pictured here.

Lory and I do a wide range of exercises; she's always changing it up. Her philosophy is that you need to cross train because the body responds differently when you introduce new exercises. It's like every time when you change your shampoo and hair products, your hair acts better. Exercise, like skincare, should be changed seasonally. No need to use a hydrating cleanser in the heat of the humid summer, go for an anti-aging, fruit based gel cleanser for ultimate performance. The same is true for exercise. In the summer months we create outdoor exercise programs, such as swimming, hiking, rowing, kayaking, working these muscles at the beach, and digging into the sand. Do things that you can't do in the winter months. Save the winter for skiing, snow shoeing, hiking, and take advantage of your indoor time to be especially reflective in your yoga practice. I believe that we dress by the seasons, we eat by the seasons, we alter our skincare by the seasons, and we should choose our exercise by the seasons too.

"Age like wine, not like milk."

Women always ask me if there are any exercises that truly help sagging necks. While I focus on exercising below the neck, the face and neck muscles also need exercise to stay fit, firm, and beautiful. I absolutely do not want to have a turkey neck. While it doesn't happen overnight, there are exercises that can help you to achieve a more youthful neck and jowls. Lory has been amazing at finding new exercises.

My Favorites Neck Toning Exercises:

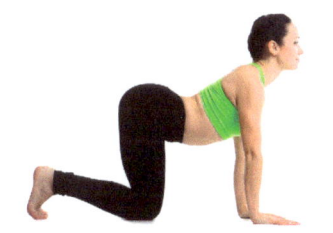

1. Go into tabletop position, as you're pushing up into cow pose, open your mouth, let go and put out your tongue and stretch your neck, and then come back to neutral. This is effective in reducing jowls and adds definition to a sagging jawline.

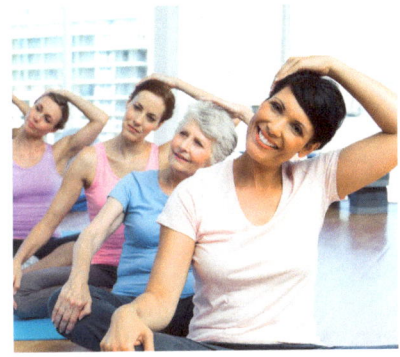

2. Side neck stretch – Sit in a chair or stand. Sit on your left hand, then bring your right hand to your left side of your head and pull towards your right ear. Then switch to the other side.

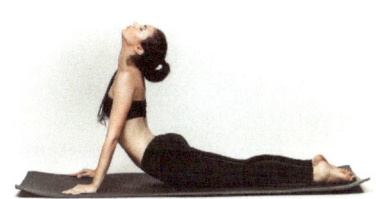

3. Get into up dog position – Lie on the floor, on your stomach and lift yourself up on your forearms, with your elbows positioned under your shoulders. Push up so that your body is in a reverse C position and tilt your chin out. Hold for several seconds and then repeat.

Beauty Exercise Tips:

• Wear sunscreen
• Wear a hat
• Stay well hydrated
• Use detoxifying toner to remove toxins after workout
• Don't exercise with makeup on your face

Stay Well Hydrated When Exercising

It should come as no great surprise that sweating and improving blood flow is good for your skin. Your skin is the largest organ for detoxification, and sweating not only helps regulate body temperature; it also helps eliminate toxins. Improved blood flow, in turn, helps shuttle oxygen and nutrients to your skin, which is key for beautiful complexion.

The Fourth Essential Element for Living Beautifully

Eat to stay and look young

Good nutrition is an essential part of being and staying healthy. By combining healthy eating with exercise; you can reach and maintain a healthy weight, reduce your risk of diseases, like heart disease and cancer, enhance your emotional well-being and reduce facial wrinkles. Reduce your wrinkles by eating right. The meals shown here are actual meals that I've cooked. Pardon me for their less then professional appearance. I cooked them in my kitchen and shot them on my iPhone.

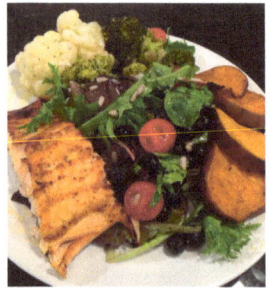

I love food, tastes, textures and will try almost anything. My father's family was in the food business for years and I studied cooking at the French Culinary Institute in New York City, during my years on Wall Street. In fact as a trade off, I taught my exercise trainer, Lory to cook and she would help sculpt my body. We've both benefited. What we have learned the most is how to improve our eating and exercise habits and to enhance our youthfulness. We look and feel great.

There are more and more studies that show that avoiding diets high in fat and sugar helps to reduce wrinkles. High fat and sugar foods slow down cell turnover and that means skin cell turnover too. Remember, as you age, your skin cells turn over more slowly. So, if you can avoid the foods that slow them down, you want to do that. And, if you can eat foods that increase our skin cell turnover, then you want to do that as well. It's when your skin cells are turning over the fastest that your skin looks the most radiant. The combination of cells turning over faster like constantly exfoliating, combined with eating foods that increase the internal skin cell turnover makes for the most gorgeous and youthful skin.

"Good people, good food."

My "must" avoid food list is pretty simple. I try to stay away from fried foods, artificial sweeteners, foods with labels that I don't understand the ingredients, and I avoid goopy desserts. And, while I do love both dairy and red meats, I rarely indulge. I eat with the goal of reducing toxins with food that are high in antioxidants. I do this to increase my skin cell turnover, not just for my face, but also for my whole body. I want to constantly flush out toxins and take in foods high in antioxidants.

Pretty in pink...

I started with a liquid mineral makeup and as I was blending, I added a touch of a tinted moisturizer for both a creamier finish and a pinker shade.

For her lips I chose red, because Gail H is all about red lips. She works long hours in both the fashion world and in real estate and she needs her look to hold up, and she knows that all reds are not created equal. I choose a long-lasting, liquid lipstick for her, and lined her lips with a deep berry touch lip liner.

To highlight her cheeks, I applied my **Bronze & Blush Face Lift Technique**. I applied bronzer under her cheekbones, under her chin, under her jaw, and over her neck area. Then I blended a pink gel blush just at and above her cheek area. I like the way a gel blush gives a luminous glow.

For her eyes I chose pinks and brown shadows using **the Side "V" Eye Shadow Technique** and one layer of eyeliner.

- **LINE** – Apply a brown liner on the top and add just a tiny bit at the bottom
- **LID** – Apply a light shade of pink eye shadow
- **"V"** – Apply a rose pink shade of eye shadow in the "V"
- **GEL LINER** – Apply black liner on the top only
- **MASCARA** – Apply black mascara to top lashes only.

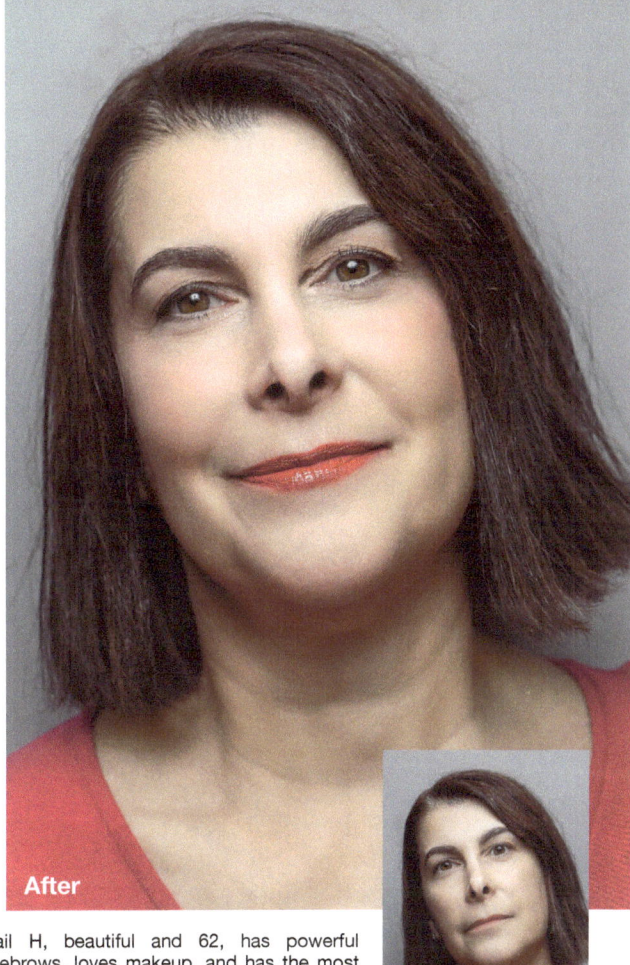

After

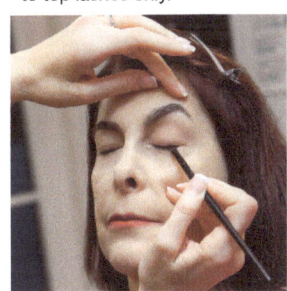

Before

Gail H, beautiful and 62, has powerful eyebrows, loves makeup, and has the most radiant skin. She takes good care of herself. I know this for sure, as I see her regularly in our studio for facials and anti-aging peels. You'd have to look really hard to find any skin discoloration on her. Her complexion is near flawless, even without makeup.

So the challenge for me, is how do I bring sparkle to a woman who already has both great brows and great skin? The answer is pink. I'm going to surround her eyes in browns and pinks, her cheeks in pink-- let's see if that adds a sparkle.

Thank You! Loved the evening as a chance to be with other women my age and see them transformed before my eyes into beauties. Their outer beauty reflected their inner beauty, which has been molded by life experiences. This point has been overlooked by society which is obsessed with the young and their skin deep beauty giving no regard as to what is coming from within.

I'm glad you're using the photos to show there still is beauty in aging women. When you become your best self, people take notice of you and listen to your wisdom. Makeup and skincare have the power to make a difference to women at any age, but especially as they grow older. You know this better then anyone!

Gail H.

Planning a meal does require some thought and imagination. Think of all of the foods with beautiful colors... Orange foods, reds, greens, yellow. It's these foods, mostly fruits and vegetables that are high in vitamin A and beta-carotene, all of which increase cell turnover for healthier skin. I'm an artist, I think in color. When I'm preparing meal, I think about what my plate will look like when it's all put together. It's a bit like making up a woman's face. I have already envisioned how I am going to apply a woman's makeup as soon as she has sat in my chair. I do the same with cooking. A well-styled plate to me is about ¾ vegetables to ¼ protein and the colors and textures look great together.

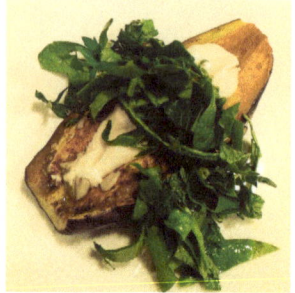

I usually start with my protein or my main vegetable dish. So, if I'm making tilapia, I have to figure out what can I put with it so the plate will look pretty and heighten the tilapia flavor? Or, if I'm making roasted Moroccan Eggplant, I have to decide what to accompany this dish to enhance both its look and its flavors?

I'm pretty sure this method of meal planning rubbed off on my twins. When they were young, we would gather around the kitchen island doing homework and cooking dinner, I would ask for their help with dinner. I'd say, "We're having grilled salmon for dinner, what else should I put on the plate to look pretty with the salmon?" My daughter might suggest steamed carrots and my son would say "No... too much orange. Let's choose something green like maybe string beans or spinach." Then my daughter one would pipe up and say, "I want broccoli. That will look pretty." This banter was very cute. I'd get all sorts of suggestions of different colors and textures from vegetables to grains. It was a good way to get them involved and creative. Their favorite meal was still macaroni and cheese, which just made me cringe.

"Be with someone who brings out the best in you, not the stress in you."

Diet does affect your complexion, your skin, and your youthfulness. It may not be medically proven, but there are many articles written about herbs and their anti-aging effects. Some herbs are believed to help boost the body's immune system, improve cell reproduction, and increase blood circulation. I incorporate certain herbs into my diet because they can be added as a spice and flavor to foods I'm already eating and they might even help to keep me younger.

Here is my list of foods that I think are skin-enhancing. I usually try to base my meal planning and dining around:

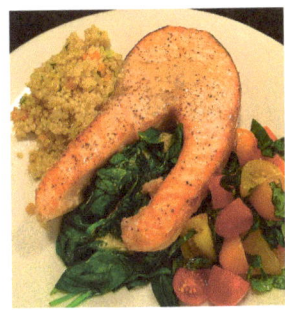

Green Tea
Tomatoes
Kale
Salmon
Oysters
Edamame
Olive Oil
Walnuts

Eggs
Broccoli
Pumpkin
Sunflower Seeds
Red Bell Peppers
Lemons
Dark Chocolate
Carrots

I believe that there are youth-enhancing herbs. I try to incorporate most of these into my daily diet. Maybe they are youth-enhancing, but at the very least they are flavor-enhancing:

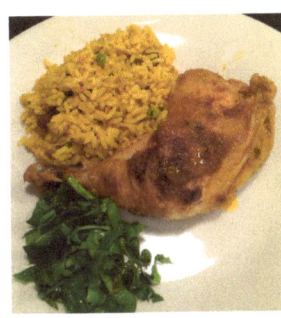

Cumin
Cloves
Cardamom
Cinnamon
Curry
Ginger
Turmeric
Cayenne

What you eat and drink should help your skin cells stay hydrated. Skin that is hydrated is generally more plump, firmer, and less likely to sag or wrinkle. Make sure you consume enough liquids, and I don't mean wine or coffee. Keeping hydrated helps you tighten your facial skin. Water is the best choice, but you can also drink non-caffeinated tea, and natural, non-sugar juices. Do I follow the 8 cups a day rule? I don't know exactly. I start my day with a large water bottle in my hand and when it's empty I grab another one, or refill it. I always have a glass or two of water by my bedside. Water is always my choice. I do drink red wine and occasionally caffeinated coffee or teas, knowing full well that they may dehydrate my skin slightly.

Red wine does have its benefits. I'm sure you've heard about resveratrol, an ingredient that is found on the skin and vines of red-wine grapes. Some people say this little chemical compound in red wine may be the reason that French women never get fat. It seems, at least to American women, that French women indulge in all of the things that we desperately try to avoid: pastries, real butter, cheese at every meal, red meat, red wine, and cigarettes – and they still mange to stay trim and youthful even into menopause. To top it off, French women have a lower incidence of heart disease than American women. Many studies credit resveratrol with their luck. I liked a daily glass of red wine, before I learned of resveratrol, but I insist on it now. By the way, you don't have to drink the wine. It is available in supplements.

Lets talk supplements and vitamins

I believe supplements can be beneficial, but the key to vitamin and mineral supplements is eating a balanced diet. Food contains thousands of fibers and phytochemicals that work together and cannot be duplicated with a pill or a cocktail of supplements. Before taking any vitamin and mineral supplements, talk to your physician or nutritionist about your personal dietary plan.

What's on the supplement menu? I am not the best pill taker, so I'm a drink your supplements kind of girl. I use a plant-based probiotic mix as my base and add it to raw kale, spinach, parsley, lemon, ginger, apple and whatever raw vegetable I have in my refrigerator, along with a large dash of cardamom, cinnamon, coriander, cumin, curry, nutmeg, and turmeric. I also chew a baby aspirin every day; I hear that keeps your heart in check and can ward off heart attacks in women (talk to your doctor). I am a fan of FABOVERFIFTY™ and they have published this as the short list of vitamins needed for women 50+: Multivitamin, Fish Oil, Calcium, Magnesium, Resveratrol, and CoQ10.

"Remember, no makeup transformation can give you everything that you desire. – It's impossible.
It's like saying that after a wonderfully satisfying dinner that you won't wake up hungry. But, we do.
That's why there's breakfast."

Dood & Janet

Rejuvenating Janet...

By the time Janet joined us for our makeover party, she had already put in a 12-hour day at the office and commuted an hour each way. Needless to say, she was exhausted. My challenge was to wake up this tired executive lady and show off her spectacular blue eyes.

I used a refreshing toner to remove the day's residue; then, a tightening serum and liquid mineral makeup. I used the attached brush for blending on her face, under her chin, and over her entire neck in order to lengthen and elongate.

Janet's Brows and Eyes: Like so many women, Janet's brows have thinned. I filled and enhanced her eyebrows using the brow filler in taupe. Once I prep a woman's skin, apply whatever tinted moisturizer, BB cream or foundation I'm going to choose and figure out what's best for her eyebrows, that's when I stand back and access what makeup look I'm going to do.

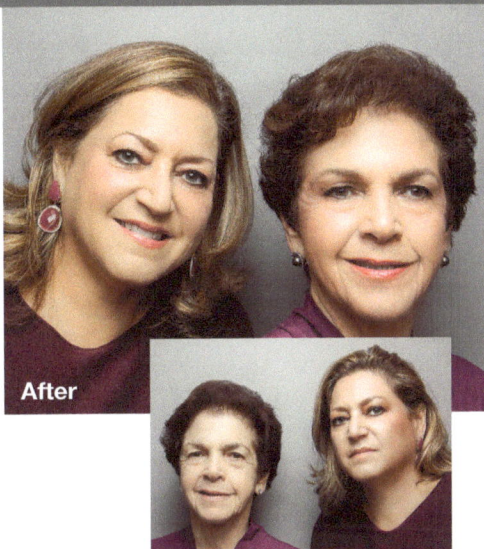

After

Before

Janet's been my friend and a client since before I created Faces Beautiful®. So suffice to say, I've done her makeup too many times to even count. For Janet's eyes and cheeks, I used the exact same colors and technique as I did for Dood. I only added in a dark blue eyeliner in her inner water area of her lower lids. For both of their eyes, I used shades of plum eye shadows using the Reverse Nude Eye Shadow Technique and extra layers of gel eye liners.

- **LID** – Use a dark plum eye shadow
- **CONTOUR** – Use shades of rose eye shadow to contour the eyelid
- **LINER** – Apply black eyeliner both on the top and bottom
- **GEL LINER** – Apply black liner on the top and add dark blue liner in the inner water area of the lower lids
- **MASCARA** – Apply mascara to top and bottom lashes.

For Janet's lips, I took into consideration the fact that Janet is not a big lipstick girl. She prefers gloss and pale colors. So after applying her light plum lip color, I lightly traced the outside of her lips, just for a bit more definition with a spice colored lip liner.

At our makeover party, a funny thing happened. I had invited Janet's mother, Dood to join us. I had done Dood's makeup hours earlier in the evening. And, so I decided to do a little experiment. I looked over to them and noticed that coincidently they were both wearing tops in the berry/plum family. An idea popped in my head. I would do Janet's makeup exactly the same as I had done her mother's. I used the same colors and the same techniques. Considering that they don't look alike, don't have the same shaped faces, not even the same coloring, I think it worked out pretty well. Janet is 58 and her mother is 81. They both look great! So pretty. Like mother, like daughter...!

Thanks again for including me in the colorful and wonderful women's night out. My mantra for women is that beauty is found at every age. I know we say that age is just a number, but we have to believe and practice it. It's essential, as you know, to communicate the importance of confidence to look one's best at any age and stage. Amazing connections and conversations can happen so easily when women get together. Men really miss out on that! Alas, there's always football!

Dood

I love watching you look at my face as a blank canvas and try to figure out what you see through your artistic eyes. I get such a thrill when you finish, smile and hold your breath as you hand me that big mirror... the reveal...

I've never been disappointed with the results and aspire to copy the look on my own.

Last night you chose my Mom and me to be made up and photographed together. You did the same application on both of us and because we have different coloring it gave us an individual to coordinated look. You had the vision and made it come alive! That's a remarkable talent.

To me, every woman that participated had a beautiful face and we spanned from mid 50's up to 80! I dare anyone to guess an age! Beauty starts from the inside and makeup enhances what we all have.

Janet

ENERGY

The Fifth Essential Element for Living Beautifully

It's About How You Feel...

We've talked about the 4 E's. And, they are all important to helping us achieve our most youthful look. It's important to exfoliate, eat right, exercise often and to know how to emphasize the beauty of your eyes. But, I feel that the most important part of enhancing your youth is your energy. Beauty starts on the inside. Positive energy is absolutely going to keep you young and radiant.

So what do I mean by energy? I like to think of energy as anything that invokes a reaction inside you. It's anything that makes you feel, makes you think, dream, or react and others can feel this energy too. Think about how you feel after you've watched a great movie, or entranced by a book, or smile every time you hear your favorite songs.

Having positive energy is absolutely essential to your youthful appearance. I wish it were simple to just feel good every day and look amazing. But, life usually gets in the way of feeling that positive energy everyday. How could it not? Life always throws us curveballs. Things go wrong, life is challenging. Whether you are managing career issues, conflicts at work, children who need you or don't need you, aging parental concerns, illness, and death, the list of complex experiences that challenge you in your lifetimes is endless. So how during all of these are you supposed to have this so-called positive energy so you can "look" good? I subscribe to two old quotes that form my mantra.

> ## "Choose to smile when you're having a bad day."

Fake It Until You Make It

This is the mindset I adopt on the days when I just feel "blah". You know these days. The days when emotionally we just feel beaten, but the march must go on. It's on those days, I drag myself out of bed, get to the gym 15 minutes earlier to sweat just a bit more and spend an extra 15 minutes getting ready. I take the extra 15 to more carefully apply my makeup, to blow out my hair better and to choose a cuter outfit. Why take more time on these 'Oh my God I just feel like crap' days? Because, if I can increase my endorphins and enhance my look, then I might just actually feel better later in the day. Or, maybe someone will see me and give me that much-needed compliment on my down day. You know, I just fake it until I actually make it.

When Life Gives You Lemons, Make Lemonade

Or, as my friend Marla says, make vodka and lemonade. I'm a pro at making lemonade – lemon chicken, lemon tarts, and lemon martinis. We all have a story. I mean really? I've certainly had my share - failed marriages, economic recessions, mean girl episodes, just to name a few. What I've really learned and I want to share with you is how I fill my emotional cabinets with healthy ingredients to keep me filled with positive energy.

Take music, for example. How does your favorite song make you feel? If you don't know what I'm talking about, dig into your iTunes or scroll through your Pandora playlist right now and put on a song you love. Take a break from reading this, close your eyes for a moment, and recognize what you're feeling. Music is one of the most powerful and recognizable forms of energy. For me music is an easy way to shift your energy quickly. I can't work with bad music and I can't work in quiet. When I'm creating a makeup look for a client, I need pop music. I have a very wide collection of music across many genres, but makeup music has to pop.

Positive energy is contagious. You can catch this from others and they can feel it in you. That's why you look good when your energy is good. How can you obtain energy in a positive way? I'll share with you my secrets to keeping positive energy flowing.

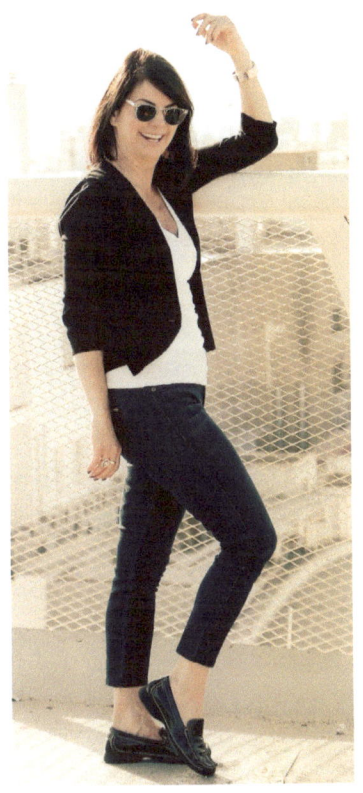

My favorite energy comes from laughter. Did you know that laughter keeps you young? Its true. And, it's no secret. Researchers have proven that laughter improves blood circulation — to the head and to the heart. Laughing is good for you. A good laugh every day improves your mood, improves your physical health and improves your emotional health. Laugh therapy has even been proven to help cure cancer and chronic illness.

Laughing heartily and uncontrollably provides a physical release. Stress hormone levels are reduced and levels of healthy hormones are increased. Your body's immune system improves with the release of endorphins, those natural 'feel-good' chemicals. It's hard to feel anxious or sad when you are having a good laugh. Muscles are exercised including the diaphragm, the abdomen muscles and the shoulders. Blood circulation is increased for all major body organs including the brain. Laughter even provides some exercise for the heart. And, the increased blood circulation stimulates your facial muscles, so you'll look better too.

Laughter is distracting from life's daily problems and worries. When laughter endorphins reach your brain, stress levels are automatically reduced. You relax and as you relax you recharge. You start to feel good and your mind clears.

> **"Happiness is the key to success. If you love what you are doing, you will be successful."**

My favorite way to create laughter is a watch a favorite funny movie. Everyone who knows me knows that I love movies and love to laugh. Some say my laugh is infectious. I certainly hope so. Here is a short version of my classic go-to laugh movies: *Bridget Jones Diary, Legally Blonde, How to Lose a Guy in 10 Days, White Chicks, The 40 Year Old Virgin, Billy Madison, There's Something About Mary, M*A*S*H, The Blues Brothers, My Cousin Vinny, Blazing Saddles, The Jerk* and my list continues.

If movies aren't your thing, then find some other ways to create laughter. It truly is good for your mind, your soul and your youth. Laughter fits in perfectly with my "fake it till you make it" mantra. That means just start laughing. Go to a comedy show, hang out with funny people, laugh at yourself, do something silly, be spontaneous, laugh at life's frustrations, laugh at your parents, your children, your ex, your pets. In fact, if you have children or pets, you might find that spending more time with them creates an environment that allows you to unwind and laugh more. Kids and pets are not filled with adult anxieties and they are naturally sillier and find humor in life that most adults are just too busy to notice.

I can't tell you exactly how to have good energy, but you can tell yourself. You already know all of the things that you like and the experiences that make you feel good. Maybe its best for you to make a list of your special experiences and use it as a guide as you learn to become energized from a wider variety of things. These are my two lists to positive energy. First is my what do list and the second is my think about list.

> **"What you desire is deliberately placed out of reach so that you can become the person it takes to obtain it."**

> **"A few nice words can brighten a person's day far more than you realize."**

What I do to bring positive energy into my life:

- Listen to music
- Exercise with my favorite trainer
- Do yoga
- Cook a big family dinner
- Go dancing
- Read with my book club
- Go into in the sunshine for 10 minutes
- Go to a gourmet food market
- Solve other people's problems
- Spend time with family and friends
- Stay busy
- Stay away from negative people
- Say thank you every day for my loved ones and all of our good health
- Be generous and share my love

What I *think* about to bring positive energy into my life:

- Remind myself of my wonderful qualities
- Appreciate this moment
- Forgive myself from all the things that I didn't do "right"
- Be grateful for my good health
- Recognize and appreciate the good health of my loved ones
- Focus on circulating positive ideas
- Visualize positive ideals
- Recall other people's reaction to my positive energy
- Think about what I want to feel in life
- Reflect back to those feel good experiences
- Focus on the things in life that make me feel good
- Believe in happy endings
- See my dreams fulfilled

Now It's Your Turn

Now it's your turn. It's time to incorporate these ideas into your life. One of the first things I encourage women to do is to find and pursue your passion. Through discovering your passion, you will hear your soul sing and your spirit smile. If you've already discovered your passion, consider yourself very lucky. If you haven't, you will as long as you seek it out.

> ## "Always remember that your present situation is not your final destination."

Life happens when you're ready to embrace it. Get out there and try something new, do something new, meet someone new and add my Five Essential Elements for Living Beautifully to your daily practice. Surround yourself with those who lift you up, support you, and inspire you. Having your personal sisterhood and professional network will help you to face obstacles and challenges that sometimes feel too large and daunting to deal with on your own. I don't know that I would have persevered in my career if it weren't for the constant support from my close girlfriends. Building my business has been very challenging, as times downright near impossible, especially during the last recession. Few of us would be where we are without the support of those who believed in us; and as women, we need to support each other to become the women we are meant to be. I am very thankful to all of those who support and inspire me.

Practicing my five E's will help enhance your positive energy. And, the world around you will feel it and respond more positively to you. My five Essential Elements: Exfoliate, Eyes, Exercise, Eat and Energy will make you feel and look better, more beautiful, and more confident; overall filling you with a newfound positive, fresh energy. And for that moment, the world is smiling at you.

The Five Essential Elements for Living Beautifully:

I hope my book has given you lots of tips on how to help you look fabulous, slow the aging process and maintain your everlasting youthful beauty. Your five E's should be a part of your every day life. Integrate who you love, how you live, and what you do.

1.   **Exfoliate** away your life's experiences that are over.
2.   **Eyes** - Open your eyes to all that lie ahead of you.
3.   **Exercise** your ability to make good choices.
4.   **Eat** to satiate your sensations, not to fill your holes.
5.   **Energy** - Your energy is contagious. Make it feel good.

I'm a very visual person. I believe it you can see it, you can be it or do it. By visualizing how you feel or how you want to feel, you can make the laws of attraction work for you. Many people, including myself create vision boards to help them fine tune and visualize what they are dreaming about and what it is they want from life. Visualization is one of the most powerful mind exercises you can do. Olympic athletes have been using it for decades to improve performance.

If you want to create a visualization board, concentrate on how you want to feel. Certainly you can include things you want, but the more your board focuses on how you want to feel, the more it will come to life. I do actually start with a board, like a poster board or a cork board and I print out pictures that feel right and I might add inspirational sayings, stickers or pictures I cut out from magazines. My boards incorporate my personal life and my career. Think about your goals in relationships, career and finances, home, travel and personal growth.

Here's an example of some things I include on my vision board:

- Pictures of my children – my ultimate pride and joy
- A few special friends, I love the gift of my support system
- FB logo – I want my clients to all feel good energy for my brand
- My old FB logo – a reminder of how far I have come, so I'm not upset about where I am not yet
- A few pictures from some special occasions – to remind me how enjoyable they were and how I want to be invited to many more special events
- A travel picture with my man – I so enjoy traveling and want to do much more
- Family holiday picture – traditions are so important
- Pictures making clients up – I love being in that mode
- A FB brand shot – focusing me on making beauty convenient for women
- A new FB product picture – focusing me on bringing it to the market
- A food picture – cooking, eating, food shopping all great passions
- A picture of a room I decorated that brought me lots of pleasure

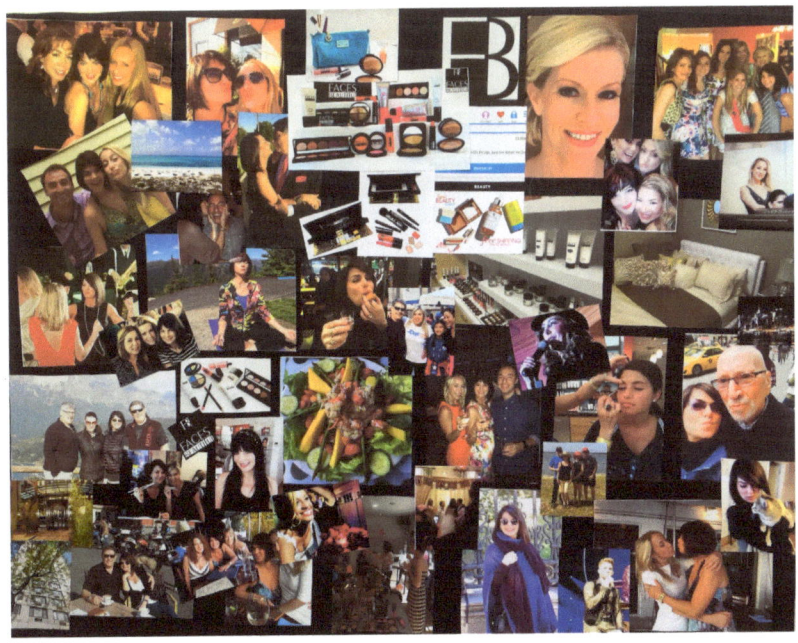

About Gail...

The path that launched me into the world of beauty as an artist, product designer, cosmetics manufacturer, and retailer, was a rather circuitous process. I started oil painting classes at age five, which was the only extracurricular activity my mother allowed. Fast forward to graduation from the University of Maryland's School of Business, which led to a 12-year journey as an institutional broker and on Wall Street. This experience was creatively stunting, but provided practical financial training, and as an oil trader, a comprehension of petroleum components that unfortunately often found its way into cosmetic products.

Then one day, bicycling home from my job at a hedge fund, I was hit by a car. On route to the hospital in the ambulance, I suffered a claustrophobic episode, leading to the realization that I was utterly unfulfilled in an uninspiring, uncreative job. The bike crash was my "aha" moment resulting in my departure from Wall Street.

After a brief hospital stint, I became active in parenting groups, co-authored a parenting book, and started a beauty business. In 2000, I launched FACES Beautiful®, a one-stop beauty retail concept store, online store and vertical cosmetics brand. This brought me in contact with a diverse clientele of actors, musicians, models, writers, CEOs, society persona, and mostly lots of everyday women.

My calling started with a fixation on eyebrows, and the art of brow shaping and filling is how I launched into the beauty world. *If the eyes are a window into one's soul, then the eyebrows are a skylight to one's beauty.* Through the brows, a woman's facial beauty can be totally transformed.

When I first meet someone, my gaze goes from their outfit to their face, and I often find myself reshaping women's poorly executed brows. I cringe when I encounter unruly, over-waxed brows, and can't help but wince at angry brows that make women look mad. But with the proper brow treatment, a woman can be made to look younger, more sophisticated, glamorous, alluring, and elegant.

Despite intense competition in the beauty industry and trying economic conditions, I have managed to survive and thrive, owing to a great upbringing, an overactive right brain, and my Wall Street experiences. My brand and store, FACES Beautiful®, has been an eight-time recipient of Best of Westport and winner of the 2016 Spectrum Award, earning a 5 star rating. I feel especially gratified to have received the 1st place beauty award for the "best foundation" by *Bella Magazine* for my "Brush-On" Liquid Mineral makeup, a must-have product in every woman's clutch. My work has been featured in *New Beauty, ELLE Canada, PARADE Magazine, The Examiner, Bella Magazine, VIV Magazine, Westport Magazine, Fairfield Magazine,* and SheKnows.com. I have been recognized by the National Association of Professional Women.

My career trajectory is more exciting than I ever anticipated, and has produced three epiphanies I'd like to share: 1) don't mold yourself based on what you think others want you to be, 2) stand by your intuition, and 3) follow your passion, even if sounds crazy to others.

My passion is about appreciating and respecting women through beauty. My niche is teaching women my quick, easy-to-do-makeup techniques to create everything from an "everyday look" to that "special look." To that end, I lead empowering workshops that teach women how to look and feel confident just by enhancing one's natural beauty. My makeup manuals are devoted to teaching women not just how to look more beautiful, but also how to feel beautiful by inspiring self-confidence and smiling more.

I thought you'd like to see what my transformation looks like too. Seems only fair.

I recognize that women want to know what the experts know, buy the products we buy, and recreate professional results in your own home. My goal is to show you high-performance, easy to use products that enable you quick results and fulfill your beauty agenda. For me, it has never been just about the makeup, it is about making faces beautiful and making our lifestyles easier.

Be beautiful,

Gail Sagel

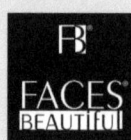

PRODUCT GLOSSARY:

Karen:
SuperWear Makeup Remover
Papaya Enzyme Toner
Natural Velvet Moisturizer
Radiant Beige Brush-On Liquid Mineral Makeup
Precious Naturals Five Shades of Eyes
Noir Gel Eyeliner
Voyage Gel Eyeliner
Lush Mascara
Persimmon Mineral Blush
Matte Sheer Lip Color - Colorado 303
Luscious Cranberry Lipshine

Carol:
Skin Transforming Serum
Healthy Nude Brush-On Liquid Mineral Makeup
The Nude Palette
Ramona Mineral Matte Bronzer
Naughty Pink Mineral Blush
Gold Candle Glow
Red Carpet Lipstick
Bordeaux Gel Lip Liner

Lindsey:
Skin Transforming Serum
Radiant Beige Brush-On Liquid Mineral Makeup
Cameo Glow Mineral Sheer Tinted Moisturizer
The Nude Palette
Lush Mascara
Noir Gel Eyeliner
Voyage Gel Eyeliner
Iced Violet Lipstick
Skinny Dip Gloss

Tami:
Hydrating Refresher Toner for Dry Skin
Skin Transforming Serum
Healthy Nude Brush-On Liquid Mineral Makeup
Monochromatic Five Shades of Eyes
Cinnamon Sugar Gel Lip Liner
Barely There Lip Shine
Lush Mascara

Rivers:
Hydrating Refresher Toner for Dry Skin
Reparative Moisture Cream
Porcelain Mineral Sheer Tinted Moisturizer
Gold Candle Glow
Shimmy Shimmer Five Shades of Eyes
Noir Gel Liner
Lush Mascara
Harmony Light Mineral Bronzer
Cantaloupe Mineral Blush
Prima Lipstick
Bordeaux Gel Lip Liner
Skinny Dip Gloss

Gail H:
Healthy Nude Brush-On Liquid Mineral Makeup
Cameo Glow Mineral Sheer Tinted Moisturizer
Blush Nude Five Shades of Eyes
Noir Gel Liner
Lush Mascara
Harmony Light Mineral Bronzer
Grace Pressed Mineral Gel Blush
Razz Dance Liquid Lipstick
Bordeaux Gel Lip Liner

Pam:
Porcelain Mineral Sheer Tinted Moisturizer
Light Dual Action Concealer
Plum Perfect Five Shades of Eyes
Blush Nude Five Shades of Eyes
Noir Gel Liner
Symmetry Bronzer Pressed Mineral Gel Blush
Grace Pressed Mineral Gel Blush
Delaware Matte Sheer Lip Color
Bordeaux Gel Lip Liner
Blush Rose Gloss
Lush Mascara

Ellie:
Radiant Beige Brush-On Liquid Mineral Makeup
Plum Perfect Five Shades of Eyes
BlackWaterproof Liquid Pen Eyeliner
Voyage Gel Liner
Zebra Canyon Mineral Matte Bronzer
Pretty in Pink Mineral Blush
Electric Taffy Liquid Lipstick

Dood:
Hydrating Refresher Toner for Dry Skin
Skin Transforming Serum
SuperWear Brow Definer
Plum Perfect Five Shades of Eyes
Noir Gel Liner
Lush Mascara
Ramona Mineral Matte Bronzer
Fuschia Mineral Blush
Guam Matte Sheer Lip Color
Spicy Plum Lipshine
Bordeaux Gel Liner

Janet:
Papaya Enzyme Toner
Peptide Serum
Radiant Beige Brush-On Mineral Makeup
Taupe
Brow Definer
Perfect Plum Five Shades of Eyes
Noir Gel Liner
Voyage Gel Liner
Lush Mascara
Spicy Plum Lipshine
Cinnamon Sugar Gel Lip Liner

www.facesbeautiful.com

Thank you for your purchase of **FACE IT**!

If you enjoyed this book and you learned even one new tip, I would love to hear from you.

Contact me at Info@facesbeautiful.com
Write a review on Amazon.

www.ingramcontent.com/pod-product-compliance
Lightning Source LLC
Chambersburg PA
CBHW040313010626
45792CB00022B/283